DOCTORS Killed
George Washington

D0187994

DOCTORS Killed George Washington

Hundreds of Fascinating Facts from the World of Medicine

Erin Barrett and Jack Mingo

Foreword by David Colbert

CONARI PRESS
Berkeley, California

Conari Press books are distributed by Publishers Group West.

Cover Illustration: Colin Johnson
Cover and Book Design: Claudia Smelser
Author Photo: Jen Fariello

Library of Congress Cataloging-in-Publication Data

Barrett, Erin.
    Doctors killed George Washington : hundreds of fascinating
    facts from the world of medicine / Erin Barrett, Jack Mingo;
    foreword byDavid Colbert.
        p.   cm. — (Totally riveting utterly entertaining trivia)
    Includes bibliographical references.
    ISBN 1-57324-719-7
    1. Medicine—Anecdotes. 2. Medicine—Humor. 3.
    Medicine— Miscellanea. 4. Wit and humor in medicine. I.
    Mingo, Jack. II. Title. III. Series.
R705 .B326 2002
610—dc21   2001005708

Printed in the United States of America on recycled paper.

02 03 DATA 10 9 8 7 6 5 4 3

DOCTORS Killed George Washington

foreword

by **David Colbert**

editor of the *Eyewitness to America* series
and author of *The Magical Worlds of Harry Potter*

Step right up, ladies and gentlemen. This book cures all ills. Ground into a fine powder and stirred in milk, it speeds the synapses of the brain. Rubbed heartily on the site of a wound, it miraculously repairs the skin. It mends; it heals; it cures. It invigorates the senses and is a restorative to the mind.

What? You don't believe me? But every foreword to a funny book about medicine begins with the old lie that laughter is the greatest healer. Of course, some of us prefer Demerol when we're going under the knife, but if you're happy listening to an old George Carlin routine over the surgery room's loudspeakers, go right ahead. That wouldn't even come close to being as strange as some of the stuff Erin Barrett and Jack Mingo have collected here.

It's not exactly the serious side of medicine, but don't worry: If you need help passing exams, there's always a rerun of a hospital drama playing on television.

Preface

According to historians, medicine is probably humankind's oldest profession. Starting with the simple herbalism and the tribal shamanism of prehistory, the medical profession has made giant strides and great leaps in knowledge and technique, forever changing the ways in which we understand the human body and how it works. However, the *idea* of healing the body and the mind remains the same today as it did for those first doctors.

As we were writing this book, we ran into case after case of some combination of genius, observation, perseverance, coincidence, and just plain luck that came together to move medical science forward. We have to be amazed at stories like that of a milkmaid who helped a country doctor invent the smallpox vaccine, or of the doctor who used himself as a test subject in order to discover the real cause of ulcers.

Not that there weren't some wrong turns along the way. In fact, there were entire eras when the whole of medical practice could be pretty much described as a wrong turn. How else to explain the surgeons who ridiculed the idea of washing their hands before operating? Or the doctors who recommended tobacco as a cure-all? And, of course, there were George Washington's doctors, who took a mild complaint and turned it into a medical crisis, bleeding their famous patient over and over again until he died.

Reading of the folly of medicine's best minds in times past and present, we can't help but wonder what will be the reaction of future historians to our own as yet undiscovered folly. It is clear that the proper attitude toward the profession of medicine is both pride at how far we've come . . . and humility at how long it's taken to get here.

To help this process—of both pride *and* humility—let us dedicate this book to all medical professionals (and those who love them). As the poet Lord Byron prescribed: "Always laugh when you can. It is cheap medicine."

Erin Barrett
Jack Mingo

one

Medical Oddities

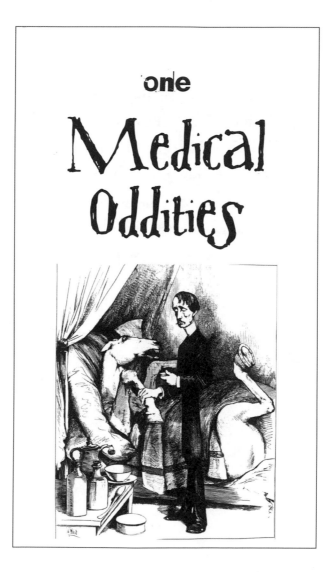

It's true that official death rates go down when doctors go on strike. For example, a recent doctors' strike in Israel saw death rates tumble by 39 percent. Yes, some drop might have come because life-threatening operations were postponed. But here's how to account for most of the drop: In reality, death goes on as normal; it's just that a strike postpones the filling out of death records.

Arteries & Science

A study found that 1 out of 4 patients diagnosed with high blood pressure in a doctor's office has normal blood pressure when measured away from the doctor's office.

A healthy human's blood pressure is about the same as a spider's.

Licorice can raise your blood pressure.

The official name for that blood-pressure measuring cuff is a *sphygmomanometer*.

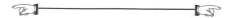

Light flickering at a rate of 10–30 blinks per second can stimulate epileptic seizures in some people. Children are most susceptible—the peak age is thirteen—and three-quarters of the victims are boys.

Culprits have included cartoons, video games, TVs with bad vertical hold, disco lights, and even the sun shining through venetian blinds.

Anybody who has given up chocolate for tofu can completely understand this: Statistical studies in the 1990s indicated that lowering blood cholesterol, while healthy for the heart, appeared to correlate to depression and deaths from suicide, violence, and accidents.

If you work with pigs, you're more likely to have your appendix operated on: two and a half times more likely if you're a pig farmer; four times if you're a pig butcher. Pigs carry the *Yersinia* bacteria, which can cause both appendicitis and a harmless intestinal inflammation that closely mimics appendicitis. As a precaution, doctors have had to operate either way, discovering only after cutting open the body whether their pig-wrangling patients have diseased appendixes or healthy ones.

Saints Preserve Us!

According to Catholic teaching, Saint Apollonia is the patron saint of dentists. Her claim to the job comes because an angry mob yanked out her teeth one by one in 249 C.E. when she refused to renounce Christianity.

Saint Harvey is the patron saint of optometrists, a little strange since he was blind from birth and was never credited with any eye-related miracles.

Pick your disease and the Catholic Church has a patron saint for it. Here are some you may wish to know about: Saint Acacius (headaches), Saint Cathal (hernias), Saint Giles (lameness, insanity, sterility, and epilepsy), Saint Drogo ("gravel in the urine"), Saint George (syphilis), Saint Catherine of Alexandria (diseased tongues), Saint Lucy (eye diseases, dysentery, and "hemorrhages in general"), Saint Hilary of Poitiers ("backward children"), Saint Servatus ("leg diseases"), and Saint Benedict (fever, inflammation, kidney disease, and "temptations of the devil").

What's the "cape doctor"? A prevailing wind in the Cape of Good Hope that locals have long believed prevents illnesses by carrying germs out to sea.

At Tokyo's Kei University Hospital, 30 percent of patients diagnosed with throat polyps claimed that karaoke singing was the cause.

There is a lot of anecdotal evidence that people are particularly irritable between 4 and 6 P.M. Here's one bit of statistical evidence: In hospital emergency rooms, more human bites are treated during that two-hour time period than in any other.

Doctors in Fiji during World War II discovered that coconut milk can be used as an emergency substitute blood plasma and that coconut fiber works better than catgut for stitching surgical incisions. But that's not all. Some South Pacific coral is so nearly identical to human bone in mineral content and porosity that it's been used by plastic surgeons to replace human bone.

Conflict of Interest: Before the 1930s, many ambulance services were operated by funeral homes.

Much turn-of-the-twentieth-century silliness greeted the invention of the x-ray. Evangelists tried to find the soul with it. A professor tried to use x-rays to transmit anatomical drawings directly into his students' heads. New Jersey considered a law to make it illegal to sell x-ray glasses designed for looking through women's clothes. For added safety, a London clothes manufacturer did a brisk business in selling "x-ray-proof undergarments" to shy ladies.

God Bless You! June Clark was a Miami teenager who had sneezed continuously for 155 days in a row. After several other approaches failed, they started giving her mild electric shocks each time she sneezed. For whatever reason, it stopped her sneezing pretty quickly.

Einstein's Brain

Last time we checked, Albert Einstein's brain is still in Wichita with the man who did his autopsy in 1955. Dr. Thomas Harvey mostly keeps it in a bottle in his office, except for the occasional outing. For example, Harvey schlepped the brain cross-country to visit Einstein's granddaughter in 1997, reuniting generations even after death.

Was Einstein's brain different from yours and mine? In the summer of 1999, a group of scientists from McMaster University in Ontario borrowed the brain from Dr.

Harvey and found that the inferior parietal region—the part of the brain that's associated with mathematics, visuals, and music—is 15 percent wider than most people's brains.

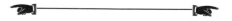

If you define obesity as being thirty pounds or more over a healthy weight, Russia's people are the most obese people in the world (25.4 percent of their citizens), followed closely by Mexico's (25.1 percent). The United States isn't far behind—about 20 percent, or 1 in 5.

Cutting & Pasting

According to the *Guinness Book of World Records,* the world's biggest gall bladder weighed twenty-three pounds and was removed from a sixty-nine-year-old woman in Maryland in 1989.

Who had the most medical operations in history? William McIlroy of Great Britain. In the fifty years before he moved into a retirement home in 1979, McIlroy had an estimated 400 operations at a hundred different hospitals using at least twenty-two different aliases. Doctors say he had an extreme case of the psychological illness

Munchausen's Syndrome, which manifested itself in a constant craving for medical attention.

Cindy Jackson—not Michael Jackson—holds the record for the most elective plastic surgery done: twenty-seven operations over a period of nine years. Born on a pig farm in Ohio, Jackson has had two nose jobs; three full face lifts; thigh liposuction; jawline, knee, and abdomen work; breast reduction and augmentation; and permanent makeup. She has spent about $100,000. And we hope she is finally happy with the way she looks.

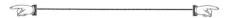

An American urologist was the buyer of Napoleon's penis in 1977. He paid $3,800, or roughly $3,800 per inch (to be fair, it was unerect). The penis was one of several body parts removed during autopsy by a team of French and Belgian doctors.

Henry VIII chopped off the head of his wife Anne Boleyn. Perhaps he should've started with other body parts first. She suffered from the condition of polymazia, meaning that she had three breasts, and had six fingers on one hand and six fingers on one of her feet.

Can your heart stand still without you dying? Sure, happens all the time in rests between beats. If you added them all together in an average lifetime, you'd find that your heart stands still for about twelve years.

Premature Burial

For about 150 years during the seventeenth and eighteenth centuries, people in Europe and America were in the grip of an obsessive fear of being buried alive. Helpful doctors came up with reassuring procedures to make sure a dead person was really dead. For example, blowing tobacco smoke up the anus with a special pipe was thought to be a solid way of separating the quick from the dead. It probably still is.

Lurid stories were spread in the popular press about premature burial. Some of them were spread by well-meaning doctors; for example, postmortem reports described corpses with their fingers chewed off—a sign, some doctors said, that the corpse awoke and was panicked and hungry enough to chew its own extremities. In reality, most or all of the cases were actually the result of rodent infestation.

Part of the problem was that doctors were not all that good at diagnosing death. In 1740, anatomist Jacques Bénigne Winslow wrote, "The onset of putrification was the only reliable indicator that the subject had died."

To avoid premature burial, Winslow suggested a series of measures to determine whether a person was really, really dead.

> The individual's nostrils are to be irritated by introducing sternutaries, errhines [things that induce sneezing and produce mucus], juices of onions, garlic and horse-radish.... The gums are to be rubbed with garlic, and the skin stimulated by the liberal application of whips and nettles. The intestines can be irritated by the most acrid enemas, the limbs agitated through violent pulling, and the ears shocked by hideous Shrieks and excessive Noises. Vinegar and salt should be poured in the corpse's mouth and where they cannot be had, it is customary to pour warm Urine into it, which has been observed to produce happy Effects.

Of course, if none of these actually produced the "happy Effects," it was time to bring out the tough love, just to make sure the presumed corpse was really dead: cutting the soles of the feet, thrusting needles under the nails, pouring hot wax on its forehead, and even—suggested one doctor/cleric—probing the anus with a hot poker. If none of these actually elicited a response, doctors assumed that they could safely pronounce the person dead.

There is no written record, by the way, of any of these methods actually reviving anybody. Too bad—we'd like to hear the reactions of the revived person awakening to the ministrations described above.

Premature Resurrection

In 1788 in New York City, eight people were killed and scores wounded in three days of rioting against doctors. And the house of one Sir John Temple was looted when the semi-literate mob misread his title and first name as "Surgeon." What set "the Doctors Riots" off? A prank by a medical student named John Hicks Jr., who terrified a boy by waving a dismembered corpse's arm at him and telling him that the arm had belonged to his mother. The boy's father and his brick-laying co-workers rushed the laboratory and, discovering mutilated corpses, wrecked the place. The civil unrest spread from there.

Grave robbing by faculty and students was very common at the time. Calling themselves "Resurrectionists," teacher-student teams would illegally stage midnight raids on local graveyards, pulling a freshly buried body out of the ground and replacing the dirt in about an hour. It became the custom among grieving citizens in some university towns to place iron bars on a grave and post an armed guard on the site for two weeks, until the body had putrefied enough to make it unusable for dissection.

The Doctors Riots sound like they should be shrugged off as a bizarre anomaly, but that's not true. Between 1765 and 1852 there were at least thirteen riots against grave-robbing medical schools in Illinois, Maryland, Massachusetts, New York, Ohio, Pennsylvania, and Vermont.

two

Medicine Marches On. . . .

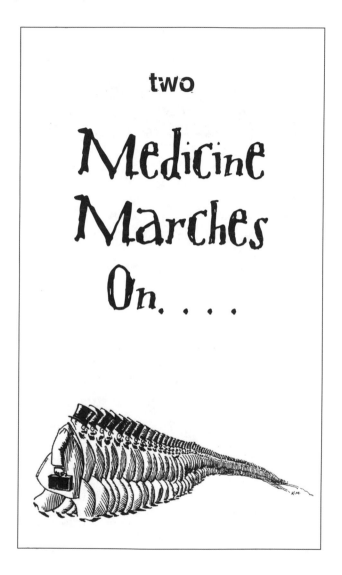

"It should be the function of medicine to help people die young as late in life as possible."

—Dr. Ernst Wunder, president of the American Health Foundation

What's the world's oldest profession? Anthropologists say health care, in the form of a tribal shaman.

Ironically, very early medicine was often as good as or better than that of more recent eras. Doctors in ancient societies had figured out sutures, poultices, resetting dislocations and fractures, splints, and the importance of cleaning wounds. They used purges, laxatives, emetics, enemas, diuretics, and a wide variety of plant extracts, at least fifty of which—including narcotics, painkillers, and digitalis—are still in use today.

The first psychotherapists may have been a priestly Greek sect called the Asclepiades. They claimed to be direct descendents of Asclepius, the god of healing.

Long before penicillin was discovered, Egyptian doctors used it without knowing it: they treated infected wounds with moldy bread.

The earliest known dentists practiced in Egypt around 3700 B.C.E.

As far as we know, Egyptians were the first who used gold for filling teeth. That was about 4,500 years ago.

The same oils, gums, and spices that Egyptian mummifiers used to preserve the dead were used by Egyptian doctors to protect wounds.

Ancient Greek doctors discovered that urine was aseptic and so used it, or a mix of wine and vinegar, on open wounds.

In ancient times, electric eels were sometimes used to give shock treatment to epileptic patients.

The ancient Hindus were skilled surgeons, and were probably the first to succeed with reconstructive surgery. They're credited with performing the first skin grafts.

Amynthas of Alexandria is credited by some with having carried out the first nose job (rhinoplasty). This was in the third century B.C.E.

How did barbers end up being surgeons in previous centuries? Blame the Fourth Lateran Council of the Catholic Church. In 1215, it forbade clerics to spill blood, so surgery was forbidden to priests, scholars, and gentlemen. Physicians continued to be considered members of a learned profession; because they had steady hands and the necessary tools, barbers and dentists practiced surgery, then considered a more menial profession.

In the 1600s, it became the height of fashion to dress up and go to an anatomy theater to watch surgeons dissect corpses. The anatomy theater in Leyden, Italy, for example, had hundreds of seats and sometimes still had standing room only crowds.

During the days when drawing and quartering was a popular punishment, anatomy students were encouraged to go to public executions to see what they could learn when prisoners were cut into four pieces and their internal organs pulled out.

One of the most successful physicians of the American colonies was not a doctor at all but a lawyer and governor of Connecticut. Since there were so few real doctors who made the trip to the New World, any educated person was expected to lend a hand. John Winthrop arrived in Connecticut in 1631 and, when he was not performing his duties as governor, developed a large medical practice that included a number of distant patients that he saw only by mail (notably including Roger Williams, founder of Rhode Island).

Doctors in Tudor-era England were expected to take up residence in a patient's house until he or she got better.

Before the germ theory took hold, most learned medical people believed that disease was caused by "miasma," a smelly gas. The fact that sewage pits, rotting carcasses, and the like—all of which really could spread disease—smelled bad was seen as positive proof of the theory.

How did doctors discover that lymph nodes act as a blood filter? It happened accidentally while doing an autopsy on a sailor. He was heavily tattooed and his lymph nodes were dyed with ink that had migrated.

Christopher Wren invented the first hypodermic needle, using a hollow feather quill and a sheep's bladder to inject a dog with opium, to no ill effect. Wren was the architect who, after the Great London Fire of 1666, designed many of the major buildings in London.

Despite the mythology, George Washington didn't have wooden teeth. He actually had four sets made from a mix of hippopotamus bone, elephant ivory, and teeth from cows and dead people. None of them worked very well, and the discomfort of his dentures is one of the reasons Washington looks so sour in his portraits. (While we're separating tooth from lie, let's do another one: Despite legend, Paul Revere never crafted a set of dentures for Washington.)

Johannes Kepler had many accomplishments as an astronomer, but he was also the first to realize that the construction of the eye inverts the images of what it sees.

The first eyeglasses were designed by Franciscan monks, William de Rubruk and Roger Bacon, in the late thirteenth century. More than four centuries later, Ben Franklin hit middle age and needed two sets of glasses, so he did the monks one better. He halved his two sets of lenses and glued the mismatched pieces together, creating the first bifocals.

Although Leonardo da Vinci sketched out the idea of contact lenses in the late fifteenth century, the first ones weren't made until centuries later. The first attempt at a glass contact lens took place in the 1880s and was designed for someone who had had an eyelid amputated. It covered the whole eye.

The first successful corneal transplant took place in 1835 and was performed by a British army surgeon stationed in India. The patient was his pet antelope. It had only one eye, and that eye had a badly scarred cornea. The donor was a freshly killed wild antelope. After the operation, the pet was able to see again; the donor didn't come out nearly as well.

"Wherever the art
of medicine is loved,
there also is a love
of humanity."

—Hippocrates

War is hell, but it often leads to medical advances. Such is the case with plastic lens implants, a result of World War II. A doctor inspected the injured eyes of a pilot who had been flying a Spitfire whose windshield had been shattered by German gunfire. The windshield was made from newfangled plastic instead of glass, and the doctor noticed that the plastic fragments did comparatively little damage. Four years after the war ended, the first plastic lens was successfully implanted into a human being.

At the time of the American Revolution, there were about 4,500 men practicing medicine in the United States, and many more women (mostly as midwives). However, only about 300 of the "doctors" actually had medical degrees.

A shotgun accident on Mackinac Island, Michigan, in 1822 led army doctor William Beaumont to the greatest single contribution toward understanding the digestion process. A young fur trapper named Alexis St. Martin took a shotgun blast to the belly, and Beaumont nursed him back to health. However, a flap of skin into the stomach did not heal, allowing Beaumont over a ten-year period to observe the workings inside, including inserting bits of food on string to check their digestion rates.

Until 100 years ago, there was no chemical test for diabetes. The only way to check for sugar in the urine was to taste it. A medical book written 500 years ago advised doctors that "it is below the dignity of physicians to do it" and suggested leaving the task to a servant or the patients themselves.

Because of advances in medicine (and possibly in weaponry), World War II was the first major war in history in which infectious diseases claimed fewer casualties than battlefield injuries.

During the twentieth century, the average American life span increased more than thirty years.

Palpitating (tapping) a patient's chest was inspired by a winemaker: Austrian doctor Leopold Auenbrugger, who was the son of a vintner. He often watched his father tap wine barrels to check the amount of wine inside and realized that listening to the sound of a chest could indicate a lot about what was going on inside it. He published his findings in 1761.

Surgeon Guido Lanfranc was inspired by violinmakers when he came up with his method of checking for skull fractures. Working in the fifteenth century, he'd have patients clasp a catgut string in their teeth. He'd hold the other end and pluck the string. A sweet clear note indicated that the skull was intact; a dull twang meant that the skull was cracked.

Sometimes scientists get the right answer for the wrong reasons. In 1779, a priest and biologist named Lazzaro Spallanzani filtered semen from amphibians to try to figure out what exactly caused conception. He discovered that semen became less and less effective the more complete the filtration was but that the residue filtered out—solids and spermatozoa—retained the power to impregnate. However, he came to the wrong conclusion: He decided that it was the mucousy solids that caused impregnation and that the spermatozoa were some sort of parasite.

Anton van Leeuwenhoek's awestruck description of the microbes he saw swimming around under his first microscope in 1642: "Hundreds of little beasties!" Leeuwenhoek not only discovered the microscope but also bacteria, protozoa, and spermatozoa. He had no medical or scientific training of any kind.

A few years after Leeuwenhoek's discovery, a colleague discovered the existence of "cells" while looking at thinly sliced wood and cork. Where the name came from: He thought that the neat rows of squares looked like the living quarters of monks.

The first stethoscope was a rolled-up sheet of paper. It was used on an obese woman whose heartbeat couldn't be heard through her layers of fat. After continually pressing his ear against her over-ample chest, Dr. Rene Läennec rolled up a sheet of paper and put his ear against one end while he pressed the other against the woman's chest. It worked! Läennec realized that this could also be a good way of handling shy patients who were reluctant to have a doctor press his ear against their breasts. He adapted his roll of paper into the device used today.

In World War I, before antibiotics, curing badly infected wounds was difficult. Doctors had great success with an unlikely source—fly larva. Sterilized maggots did a superlative job of cleaning up the ragged and infected edges, and their excretions were full of allantoin and urea, which helped keep infections in check.

The first artificial heart valve in the 1950s used a tiny plastic ball to alternately open and shut the blood flow. The only problem was that when patients opened their mouths, clicks from the valve were annoyingly loud.

The first artificial heart was made of Dacron and was implanted deep in the chest of a Texan in 1969. He died four days later.

Insulin in sufficient purity for human injection was first extracted from the pancreatic tissue of dogs in 1921. As full-scale production began, they used sheep and hogs. Finally, in 1981 scientists genetically engineered bacteria to produce genuine human insulin from nonhuman sources.

Thicker Than Water

Historians believe that the Incas may have been the first to do successful blood transfusions. What would have made the job easier is that they were all the same blood type (O positive).

1492, the year of Columbus and the expulsion of Jews from Spain, witnessed the first contemporary documented attempt at a blood transfusion. The doctor was attempting to save a dying pope, Innocent VIII. Not only did the pope die, but so did the three boys from whom the doctor extracted blood. The doctor quickly went on the lam, and blood transfusions weren't tried again for nearly two centuries.

In 1665, Dr. Richard Lower of England successfully transfused blood back and forth between two dogs using feather quills. Unfortunately, he then tried a lamb-to-man transfusion. The man died, and research into blood transfusions was abandoned for another 150 years.

In 1818, Dr. James Blondell saved a man's life with the first documented person-to-person blood transfusion. Unfortunately, because people had not yet unraveled the mystery of blood typing, his next attempts were failures. Patients died, and research ceased for another century.

Why is blood typing important? Mixing incompatible blood quickly creates a sea of red dumplings swimming in yellowish liquid, bringing on instantaneous death.

In 1900, Dr. Karl Landsteiner discovered the A, B, and O blood groups and demonstrated that blood could be successfully mixed within the same group. In 1940, he helped discover the "rh factor." What does the rh in "rh factor" stand for ? It's short for rhesus, in honor of the research monkeys in whose blood Dr. Karl Landsteiner discovered these properties.

"Transfusion, transfusion
My body's just a mass of contusions
I'll never ever speed again—
Slip a gallon to me, Alan."

—*"Transfusion," 1950s novelty song
by Nervous Norvus*

The first blood bank opened in Chicago in 1937, after doctors discovered that sodium citrate would keep blood fresh and unclotted outside a donor's body.

Pioneer hematologist Dr. Charles Drew was the first to realize that blood plasma— the straw-colored liquid that remains when you remove the red cells, white cells, and platelets—would store longer than whole blood yet would be just as useful in emergency applications. He set up New York City's first blood bank in 1940. Even before the United States entered the war, Dr. Drew set up a drive to raise 5,000 units of blood plasma for England.

Dr. Drew was offended and exasperated by the U.S. military's requirement in World War II that blood be sorted by the race of its donors. For one thing, he knew that it didn't make any difference medically and that waiting for the right "race" of blood would kill soldiers and sailors. For another, military segregation, even down to blood supplies, was personally galling, since Drew was African American.

There are now about 5,000 blood banks in the United States. They're all regulated by the Federal Food and Drug Administration.

Feeling No Pain

Before surgery, ancient Egyptian doctors put their patients under by hitting them on the head with a mallet.

Oliver Wendell Holmes Sr., father of the Supreme Court Justice, discovered the adrenal gland and coined the term "anesthesia."

When anesthesia was first discovered, some ultra-religious Christians opposed it as thwarting God's will. In Scotland, Dr. James Simpson managed to still the raging controversy by equating anesthesia in surgery with the "deep sleep" in which the Bible said that God removed Adam's rib in order to create Eve.

Sir Humphry Davy was the first to recognize the intoxicating results of nitrous oxide in 1800, but he used it only for "laughing gas" parties with friends. Ether had a similar party history a few years earlier. It never occurred to Davy or anyone else to use the drugs in surgery, and eventually interest in the novelty substances dimmed.

Finally, a half-century later, a Boston dentist named W. T. G. Morton demonstrated the usefulness of the two intoxicants in front of a group of skeptical doctors. He anesthetized a tumor patient and stepped aside to allow a surgeon to operate. Dr. J. C. Warren, amazed to be working on a patient who wasn't moaning, screaming, and writhing in pain, proclaimed at the end of his operating, "Gentlemen, this is no humbug!"

Morton was not just a humanitarian, however. After his demonstration went so well, he put in an application to patent ether under the brand name Letheon. He was ruined financially by lawsuits before the courts ruled that his patent application was invalid because others had figured out the properties of ether before him.

Another dentist, Horace Wells, had tried to put on an anesthesia demonstration a few years earlier, demonstrating dentistry in front of a group of doctors. Unfortunately, he was a little stingy with the nitrous oxide and the patient began groaning in agony halfway through the operation. The doctors walked out even more convinced that surgery without pain was impossible.

Both Morton and Wells owed a debt to Samuel Cooley, who accidentally discovered the anaesthetic properties of nitrous oxide in 1844. He had gone to a popular demonstration of the gas, at the end of which the lecturer released forty gallons of it into the audience. The audience erupted into giggles and howls—Cooley, in the hilarity, stumbled and badly injured his leg without even knowing it. It was his story that inspired Wells to try using NO^2 in surgery.

three

Second Opinions

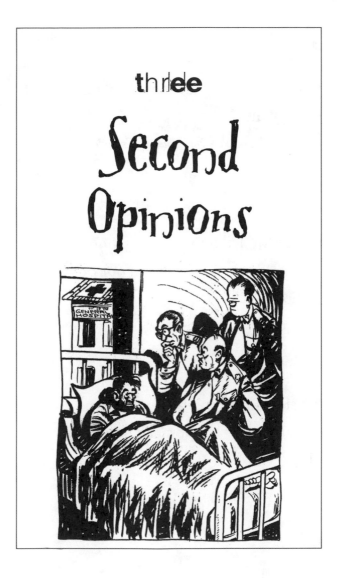

"**M**edicine is a collection of uncertain prescriptions the results of which, taken collectively, are more fatal than useful to mankind."

—*Napoleon Bonaparte, French emperor*
(1769–1821)

"**P**HYSICIAN: One upon whom we set our hopes when ill and our dogs when well."

—*Ambrose Bierce, satirist*

"**B**efore undergoing a surgical operation, arrange your temporal affairs. You may live."

—*Ambrose Bierce*

"**K**eeping off a large weight loss is a phenomenon about as common in American medicine as an impoverished dermatologist."

—*Calvin Trillin, columnist*

"**D**octors is all swabs."

—*Long John Silver, as written by*
Robert Louis Stevenson

"**O**ne of the most difficult things to contend with in a hospital is the assumption on the part of the staff that because you have lost your gall bladder you have also lost your mind."

—*Jean Kerr, humorist and author*

"**I** am dying from the treatment of too many physicians."

—*Alexander the Great*

"**S**he got her good looks from her father— he's a plastic surgeon."

—*Groucho Marx*

"**A**n ounce of prevention is worth a pound of bandages and adhesive tape."

—*Groucho Marx*

"**A** young doctor means a new graveyard."

—*German proverb*

"I firmly believe that if the whole *materia medica* could be sunk to the bottom of the sea, it would be all the better for mankind, and all the worse for the fishes."

—Oliver Wendell Holmes

"Nothing is more fatal to health than over-care of it."

—Benjamin Franklin

"God heals and the doctor takes the fee."

—Benjamin Franklin

"The art of medicine, like that of war, is murderous and conjectural."

—Voltaire

"Doctors are men who prescribe medicines of which they know little, to cure diseases of which they know less, in human beings of whom they know nothing."

—*Voltaire*

"My doctor is nice; every time I see him I'm ashamed of what I think of doctors in general."

—*Mignon McLaughlin, author*

"I got the bill for my surgery. Now I know what those doctors were wearing masks for."

—*James H. Boren, author*

"**I**f medicine is necessarily a mystery to the average man, nearly everything else is necessarily a mystery to the average doctor."

—Milton Mayer, writer
(1908–1986)

"**T**he best doctor is the one you run for and can't find."

—Denis Diderot, French encyclopedist
and philosopher (1713–1784)

"**D**octors are just the same as lawyers; the only difference is that lawyers merely rob you whereas doctors rob you and kill you, too."

—Anton Chekhov, Russian storyteller
(1860–1904)

"We have not lost faith, but we have transferred it from God to the medical profession."

—*George Bernard Shaw*

"The only way to keep your health is to eat what you don't want, drink what you don't like, and do what you'd rather not."

—*Mark Twain*

"Early to rise and early to bed Makes a man healthy, wealthy and dead."

—*James Thurber*

"After a year in therapy, my psychiatrist said to me, 'Maybe life isn't for everyone.'"

—*Larry Brown, humorist*

"Always laugh when you can. It is cheap medicine."

—Lord Byron, poet (1788–1824)

"A cheerful heart is good medicine, but a crushed spirit dries up the bones."

—Proverbs 17:22

"A rule of thumb in the matter of medical advice is to take everything any doctor says with a grain of aspirin."

—Goodman Ace,
comedy writer (1899–1992)

"Don't live in a town where there are no doctors."

—Jewish proverb

"Many serious illnesses are nothing but the expression of a serious dissatisfaction with life."

—*Dr. Paul Tournier,*
spiritual/medical author (1898–1986)

"The best doctors are Doctor Diet, Doctor Quiet, and Doctor Merryman."

—*Jonathan Swift*

"You know more than you think you do."

—*Dr. Benjamin Spock's*
Baby and Child Care

"It requires a great deal of faith for a man to be cured by his own placebos."

—*Dr. John L. McClenahan,*
medical writer

"No illness which can be treated by the diet should be treated by any other means."

—Moses Malmonides of Caldova, Jewish philosopher (1135–1204)

"Let your food be your medicine and your medicine be your food."

—Hippocrates

"Don't think of organ donation as giving up part of yourself to keep total strangers alive. Think of it as total strangers giving up most of themselves to keep parts of you alive."

—Anonymous

four

Heroes of Medicine

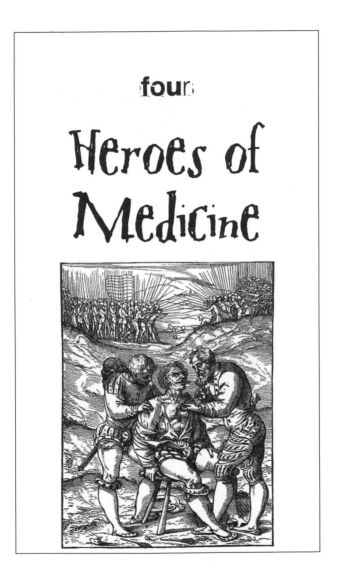

"Balto the Wonder Dog" was once a favorite running punchline of late-night host Johnny Carson. It turns out that Balto was a real dog hero. During a killer diphtheria epidemic in Nome, Alaska, in 1925, a dog team headed by Balto headed out on a 53-mile trek to deliver serum to the town in the dead of winter. The driver was blinded by snow midway through the run, but Balto found the way and saved many lives. Balto retired to Cleveland, and a grateful nation placed a statue of him in New York's Central Park. When he died in 1933, his stuffed carcass was placed in the Cleveland Museum of Natural History, where it can still be seen today.

Until Joseph Lister proved to a skeptical medical profession the value of hygiene in the late nineteenth century, surgeons bandaged surgical incisions with cloth fibers swept up from the floors of textile mills. About half of all amputation patients died as a matter of course; Lister's patients did substantially better. Regardless, Lister still had a hard time convincing the doubters. "Where are all these little beasts?" surgeon Hughes Bennet heckled during a public lecture in 1877. "Show them to us and then we'll believe in them. Has anyone seen them yet?"

Ambroise Paré, the father of modern surgery, was mocked by many of his peers because he had no academic training and didn't know Latin. During his career he invented the butterfly bandage, replaced castration for rupture patients with supportive belts and trusses, and discovered that cauterization wasn't as effective as antiseptics for stopping infections.

Researcher Alexander Fleming, haunted by his wartime experiences as a medic, investigated and wrote up penicillin's powerful antibiotic properties in 1929. He waited for the medical profession to take the ball and run with it. Unfortunately, the medical profession left the ball lying on the ground.

It wasn't until more than a decade later, on the eve of World War II, that doctors Howard Florey and Ernst Chain stumbled upon the paper in Oxford University's library and began working on making the discovery practical. All three researchers won the Nobel Prize in 1944 for saving innumerable lives.

Not a physician, but he loved to dissect things. That's how the Greek philosopher Aristotle became known as the father of comparative anatomy.

The First Nurse

Pioneer nurse Florence Nightingale, even while serving in military hospitals during the Crimean War, kept a small pet owl in her pocket.

Nightingale is famous for defining nursing as we know it today. However, she actually worked only two years as a nurse. While working with patients in the Crimean War, she contracted a fever that left her a semi-invalid for fifty-four years, until her death.

Eighteenth-century French chemist Antoine Lavoisier was the scientist who discovered oxygen. As the violence of the French Revolution roiled around him, he heard tales of decapitated heads briefly showing signs of consciousness and wondered whether such a thing was really possible. Unfortunately, he got a chance to find out when he himself was sentenced to the guillotine. Lavoisier decided on one last experiment: He told colleagues, "Watch my eyes. I will continue blinking as long as I retain consciousness." The results? After the blade came down, Lavoisier's eyes blinked for about fifteen seconds before slowing to a stop.

In the early nineteenth century, Agostino Bassi was the first person to determine that a specific disease was caused by a specific living organism invading another. He had been trying to figure out the causes of muscardine, a deadly silkworm illness. While dissecting thousands of infected silkworms, he discovered the same parasite within each. The implications were not lost on him, and he spent the rest of his life trying to convince a skeptical medical establishment that most or all of plant and animal diseases were caused by parasites.

In 1547, the Italian scientist Girolamo Fracastoro declared, "Infection itself is composed of minute and sensible particles and proceeds from them." He also was ignored by the medical profession.

The first accurate, detailed anatomical drawings were done not by a medical scientist but by artist Leonardo da Vinci, who dissected cadavers and used his skill to show the cavities of the brain and illustrate the true functions of the heart's valves.

In the early 1980s, Australian gastroenterologist Dr. Barry Marshall discovered that ulcers were caused by a corkscrew-shaped bacteria he named *Heliobacter pylori.* However, when he presented his findings to infectious disease experts in Brussels, they literally laughed out loud. After all, doctors had long believed that the stomach was sterile and that ulcers were caused by stress. They knew it so deeply that doctors routinely tossed out test results showing bacteria, figuring they must be flawed or contaminated. One problem Marshall had in proving his theory was that experimental pigs and rats are immune to the bacteria. Finally, he brewed up a batch and swallowed it himself. Sure enough, two weeks later tests showed he had a shallow ulcer swarming with *Heliobacter pylori.*

Dr. Ivan Pavlov won the Nobel Peace Prize in 1904 for medicine, but it was not for his famous salivating dog/ringing bell experiments. It was for earlier work he'd done on the automatic nervous system. Ironically, this research looked very promising in 1904 when the Nobel committee was voting, but with time it turned out to be not that significant.

There was something a little secretive about Dr. James Barry. The surgeon from Edinburgh University served in military posts all over the British Empire, worked with lepers in Africa, and won the post of Inspector of the Colonial Medical Board. It wasn't until after his death in 1865 that it was discovered that he was a she named Miranda who had been impersonating a man since the age of sixteen so that she could practice medicine.

Dr. Henry Jay Heimlich told *Who's Who in America* that he sees his invention of the life-saving squeeze maneuver as a mere footnote to what he considers his *real* calling. "My ultimate goal is to promote well-being for the largest number of people by establishing a philosophy that will eliminate war."

five

In Sickness and in Health

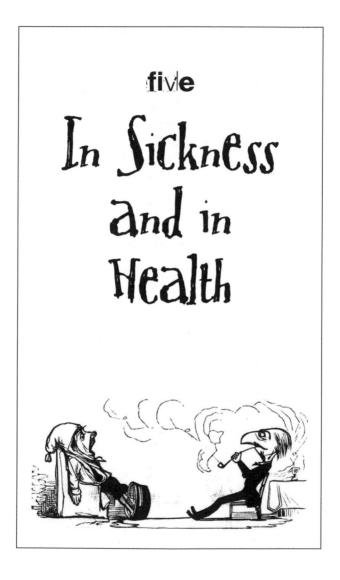

"There are no such things as incurables;
there are only things for which man has
not found a cure."

—Bernard Baruch,
financier and government advisor

Rabies viruses have to reach the brain before the disease manifests itself. Because
they travel slowly up the nerves, how quickly
an untreated victim develops rabies depends
on the distance from the bite to the brain.
A bite on the head or neck may take three
weeks. A bite on the leg may take seven.

Something You Ate? There are about
1,500 different species of salmonella,
a common cause of food poisoning.

Some are tough enough to thrive at below-freezing temperatures. For example, 224,000 Americans got sick in 1994 from a salmonella-infested batch of ice cream.

There are about 135,000 people aged one hundred or more years in the world. The United Nations predicts that there will be 2.2 million centenarians in 2050. The number has nearly doubled in the last decade, but one thing hasn't changed: the ratio of 4 out of 5 centenarians being women.

The particles from a sneeze have been clocked at a launch speed of 103.6 mph.

There are more than 100 different viruses that cause the common cold. So even though your body gets immune to whichever cold you get, dozens more are out there to give you your next cold.

According to the Centers for Disease Control, doctors prescribe annually 18 million courses of antibiotics to fight colds and 50 million courses to fight viral respiratory infections. The problem is that antibiotics don't kill viruses, so all these doses are—at best—wasteful and ineffective.

Studies indicate that people from cultures that value stoic acceptance of pain claim to experience less pain than those who are culturally allowed a greater level of emotional expression. The ever-expressive Americans are closer to the crybaby end of the scale—they report more pain during childbirth and other physical ordeals than the less-reactive Africans and Northern Europeans.

Leprosy as mentioned in the Bible was not just Hanson's Disease, as today. It referred to a number of skin diseases, including psoriasis.

Flu usually spreads from chickens to pigs to humans, mutating as it goes. The "Chicken Flu" of 1997 made medical news because it jumped directly from fowl to human, bypassing pigs.

Kids can be bad for your health. Preschool children average 6–8 colds a year. If in day care, make that 12–14 colds a year. Parents of these virus carriers average 6 colds a year, compared to 2–3 colds a year for an average non-parent.

Pleasant Dreams! Doctors have identified more than 100 sleep disorders.

"**O**ne of my problems is that I internalize everything. I can't express anger—I grow a tumor instead."

—*Woody Allen, comedian*

A research study identified sex, angry outbursts, and tennis as the triggers for 17 percent of all heart attacks.

My Boyfriend Went to America and All
I Got Was This Lousy Disease: Many historians blame Columbus and his crew for
a particularly virulent strain of syphilis that
ravaged Europe for decades after the
explorers returned from the New World.

There really was a Typhoid Mary. In early
twentieth-century New York, food worker
Mary Mallon was linked to at least seven typhoid epidemics directly infecting at least
fifty-three people, who infected another
1,300. At least three died. However, when
authorities finally tracked her down, she refused treatment and refused to stop serving
food. Finally, she was confined to Riverside
Hospital—a hospital for infectious diseases—
on North Brother Island for twenty-three
years of quarantine until her death in 1938.

Tuberculosis is an unusually ancient disease: Tubercular lesions have been found on the bones of Egyptian and South American mummies, as well as those of Neolithic humans.

A disproportionate number of people are admitted to mental hospitals during the summer months.

However, despite mythology and the source of the word *lunacy*, there has been no correlation found between a full moon and an increase in admissions to mental hospitals.

TV dramas suggest that most people who get CPR survive; however, in reality only about 15 percent do.

According to the Center for Disease Control, the ten leading causes of death are, in order:

1. Heart disease
2. Cancer
3. Stroke
4. Lung ailments including asthma
5. Accidents
6. Pneumonia or the flu
7. Diabetes
8. HIV
9. Suicide
10. Liver disease

"The first symptom in 40% of patients with heart disease is hard to deal with: sudden death."

—Dr. Michael Phelps,
inventor of the PET Scan

The number one reason Americans visit a doctor is to treat an upper respiratory tract infection.

The mortality rate for infectious disease is lowest between the ages of five and fifteen.

As many as 80 percent of people over the age of fifty suffer from arthritis.

Ninety percent of all men over eighty years old have enlarged prostates.

Thirty million men in the United States suffer from erectile dysfunction.

Modern researchers believe that some mystics, including Fyodor Dostoevsky, Saint Paul, Saint Teresa of Avila, and Marcel Proust, likely had temporal-lobe epilepsy, giving them visions and transcendental religious experiences, and feeding an obsession with matters of the spirit.

A Plague Upon You: The devastating "Spanish Flu" that appeared in 1918 wasn't really from Spain. It began in American pigs and was spread worldwide by American servicemen who had gone to fight in World War I. It killed more than 40 million people worldwide, including more than 650,000 Americans in eighteen months—more Americans than were killed in all of the twentieth century wars combined. In comparison, the Black Plague epidemic in the fourteenth century killed 25 million people in four years.

The swine flu vaccine in 1976 was based on good intentions, but it ended up causing more illness and deaths than did the disease. The disease never left the area of Fort Dix in New Jersey and caused just a few deaths; the vaccination was blamed for thousands of cases of a rare syndrome called Guillain-Barré and blamed for 25—100 deaths.

The most destructive disease through all of human history has been malaria. This year you can expect that more than 1.5 million people will die of it.

Plagues of All Nations

In 1348, casting about for a scapegoat when the Black Death swept through Europe and Asia, Swiss authorities tortured four doctors into "admitting" that they were responsible for spreading the plague. They were soon put to death, and the disease continued unabated.

Generally, the only advice physicians could give their affluent clients during a plague was to "go fast and go far" away from the cities.

When the plague swept through London in the eighteenth century, killing 12,000 people in a single week, physicians followed members of the moneyed class in fleeing the city in droves. Pharmacists—being generally less affluent and therefore less able to flee—provided the bulk of medical care to the sick and dying. The few physicians who stayed considered their lives too important to actually deal with the seriously sick; they sent assistants and surgeons into plague hospitals to care for the sick, shouting instructions up to them from the street.

Dr. Jenner's Vaccine

Dr. Edward Jenner was a country doctor in Gloucestershire, England, who noticed that people who worked near cows seemed to be immune to the plague of smallpox that was causing widespread death in Europe. Actually, that knowledge was well known among the country folk he worked with, and a milkmaid happened to clue him in. The reason the good doctor is still famous is that he took the knowledge one step further: he began deliberately infecting people with cowpox, and, sure enough, it rendered them immune to smallpox.

Research standards weren't very strict back then: To test his theory Dr. Jenner took pus from a milkmaid's cowpox pustule and inoculated an eight-year-old boy with it. Six weeks later, he inoculated the boy with deadly smallpox, but the pint-sized research subject didn't get sick.

Few American doctors believed in the vaccination theory in 1777, so it was a controversial move when George Washington had the entire Continental Army vaccinated against smallpox. He had only 4,000 men at the time and couldn't afford to lose any to sickness.

During the Franco-Prussian War (1870–1871), the Prussian army provided mandatory vaccinations. The French did not. During the months of combat, 23,400 French soldiers died of smallpox. Only 297 Prussian soldiers did.

The smallpox vaccine quickly spread across the world, nearly as fast as the disease itself. The Empress of Russia was so pleased by Dr. Edward Jenner's smallpox vaccine that by her decree the first child who got the injection took the name "Vaccinov" and was educated at the expense of the nation.

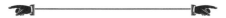

six

A Taste of Bad Medicine

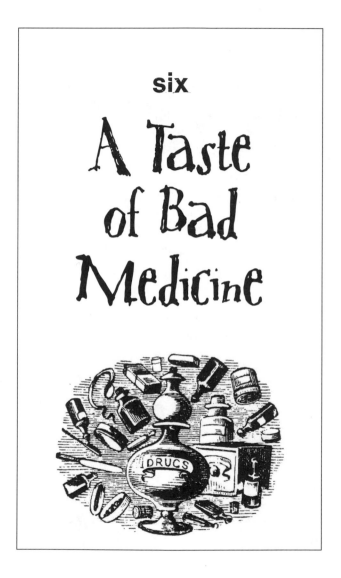

According to the Institute of Medicine, nearly 7,000 Americans are killed each year due to errors in their medication made by prescribing doctors.

More than 3 in 10 of the 3 billion prescriptions filled each year in the United States have to be rechecked with the doctor, most notably because of confusion over the doctor's handwriting.

In 1577, Spanish doctor Nicolas Monardes wrote a book called *Joyful News Out of the New-Found World,* in which he extolled a new miracle drug. The book was so influential that for two centuries, Spanish doctors prescribed the drug for dozens of illnesses, including toothaches, wounds,

stomachaches, arthritis, and bad breath.
The drug? Tobacco.

In the early twentieth century, British military doctors were justifiably concerned about infectious diseases. To fight germs, they recommended that soldiers grow mustaches and smoke cigarettes.

As late as the 1930s, many doctors treated alcoholism with a regimen of morphine injections.

Prussian surgeons in the eighteenth century treated stutterers by snipping off portions of their tongues.

Until the 1800s, most medical and dental professionals in Europe believed that tooth decay was caused by a type of worm that burrowed into the teeth. The standard treatment was to drop sulfuric acid into the cavity . . . which may not have killed the nonexistent "worm" but did destroy the nerve tissue.

In the twelfth century, Saint Bernard of Clairvaux, abbot and head doctor of the Roman Catholic Church, forbade the monks in his hospitals from studying medical texts and prohibited the use of any remedy but prayer.

According to the official reports, England's King George V died peacefully in bed minutes before midnight on January 20, 1936, after asking, "How is the Empire?" However, his doctor's notes revealed a different story when they were finally made public fifty years later. "At about 11 P.M.," wrote royal physician Lord Dawson, "it was evident that the last stage might endure for many hours, unknown to the patient but little comporting with the dignity and serenity which he most richly merited and which demanded a brief final scene. I therefore decided to determine the end." Although euthanasia was illegal in England, the doctor injected the monarch with a small dose of morphine to put him to sleep, and the king responded with his real last words— "God damn you"—before lapsing into unconsciousness. It was then that Lord

Dawson—with prior permission of the queen and the crown prince—injected the king with a lethal overdose of morphine and cocaine.

Would you like to be physician to royalty? Sure, it would have its perks, but in the Middle Ages it also had some great dangers as well. More than one doctor was put to death for not preventing a king or queen from dying.

During and after the Civil War, some of the best dentures were advertised as containing the teeth yanked out of the bodies of healthy young soldiers who had been killed in battle. It was, alas, often true.

One of the most successful though dubious medical providers of all time was John Romulus Brinkley, who'd received a doctorate from the little-known Eclectic Medical University of Kansas City. For twenty-seven years, until 1942, Brinkley made $12 million by injecting extracts made from goat testicles into aging men to cure sexual impotency and make the old goats feel like kids again.

The General's Practitioners

Like others of his time, George Washington was not immune to "miracle" medical devices. He bought a pair of quack doctor

Elisha Perkins's "Patent Tractors," a pair of metal massage bars that could allegedly cure about any disease. On the other hand, the mainstream medical establishment wasn't that much better.

Doctors killed George Washington. He called for his physicians hoping they could cure his sore throat. They went to work with vigor, bleeding him repeatedly in the hope of letting the toxins and "bad humors" out of his body. Before the day was out, Washington died.

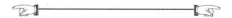

Automaker Henry Ford funded the Henry Ford Hospital, for which doctors were grateful. What they didn't appreciate, however, was that the ever-opinionated Mr. Ford liked to wander the halls and give medical advice to patients. For example, he suggested to a group of heart patients that they ignore their doctors' advice, sleep on the floor, and eat only celery.

Russian tsar Peter the Great (1682–1725) loved playing dentist and found special pleasure in extracting teeth. When his courtiers wisely stopped complaining of toothaches in his presence, Peter began randomly choosing subjects for oral inspection.

Dr. Edward Jenner, the man who conquered smallpox, came up for membership in London's prestigious College of Physicians in 1815. A problem arose: They wanted to test him in the writings of the classic medical writers. He responded that the "classics" were precisely what were holding medicine back in the Dark Ages and that conquering smallpox should be sufficient qualification. For such impudence his membership was voted down.

Long before Edward Jenner demonstrated how to make an effective vaccine, fiery preacher Cotton Mather attempted a mass inoculation against smallpox among his congregation in 1721. Pointing out the wisdom of leaving doctoring to doctors, Mather killed as many people as he protected.

Based in part on the precision practiced in his murders, some people believed that Jack the Ripper was a surgeon. One suspect was the royal physician, Sir William Gull. Another was Dr. Francis Tumblety, a reputed misogynist whose personal effects included a collection of preserved uteruses. He was hanged for murdering four prostitutes with strychnine. Legend has it that he blurted out, "I am Jack the . . ." just as the scaffold bolt was drawn.

It was a physician who was the guest of honor at the last public hanging in Scotland. More than 100,000 people turned out for the hanging of Dr. Edward Pritchard, who poisoned his wife and mother-in-law with the element antimony.

When Good Doctors Go Bad: Dr. Edme Castaing was executed in France in 1824. His claim to infame was that he was the first person to use the newly discovered drug morphine as the tool for murder, killing a wealthy patient named Hippolyte Ballet and his brother Auguste.

The wireless telegraph was used to catch a fleeing fugitive for the first time in 1910. The fugitive was Dr. Hawley Harvey Crippen. Crippen had killed his wife with an overdose of hyoscine in England and hopped an ocean liner for Canada with his mistress disguised as a boy. Crippen was recognized on the ship, and after a flurry of Morse code messages he was arrested upon arrival in Canada.

Other Really Bad Doctors: Dr. William Henry King of Ontario, who poisoned his wife in the 1850s so he could have unencumbered affairs with his patients. Dr. Morris Bolber of Philadelphia, who masterminded the deaths of thirty patients in the 1930s using untraceable poison and sandbags to the head in order to collect insurance.

Teaching hospitals seemed like a great idea in the late 1700s, and in many ways they were. However, when they first opened they brought on an epidemic of maternal deaths from puerperal fever. The problem was that for centuries surgeons hadn't seen any reason to wash their hands before surgery. That was bad enough, but it got much worse in the new teaching hospitals because surgeons would often go directly from dissecting diseased corpses to delivering babies. Some maternity wards attained an 80 percent maternal fatality rate, whereas midwife facilities next door had few or no deaths. The surgeons blamed the deaths on fumes from the cut flowers in patients' rooms. Finally, a Viennese pathologist named Ignaz Philipp Semmelweis stumbled upon a case of a male pathology assistant who died after he had infected himself with a minor scalpel cut while doing an autopsy on a woman who had died of puerperal fever. Semmelweis realized that surgeons were carrying the disease from the autopsy room to the maternity ward. After that, Semmelweis pleaded and threatened surgeons, even barricading the doors of the maternity ward to any who wouldn't sterilize his hands.

Finally in 1843, noted physician Oliver Wendell Holmes threw his considerable reputation into the battle with an article called "The Contagiousness of Puerperal Fever." It argued that Semmelweis was right and that physicians could help prevent the disease by simply washing their hands and putting on clean clothes before delivering babies. Holmes considered the article his greatest achievement in that it saved many lives. Still, it was too late for Semmelweis: ridiculed and reviled, he was eventually driven mad. He died of a disseminated streptococcal infection caused by the shackles he was forced to wear in a mental institution.

Irrational fear of cut flowers again reared its head in the 1970s when the first AIDS patients started dying and doctors had no idea what was causing it. Some physicians noticed that the men dying of pneumocystic lung infections and Karposi's sarcomas tended to have many more flowers in their room than other male patients. They seriously considered banning flowers from hospital rooms, thinking the flowers might be causing the disease.

Before Sigmund Freud became a psychoanalyst, he was a neurologist who was a pioneer in using cocaine as a local anaesthetic. Unfortunately, he didn't know it was addictive, and his overly exuberant praise of the drug as a panacea for minor pains led to a wave of cocaine addiction in Europe.

John Locke's philosophical writings helped mold the modern world's view of human rights and governments. However, his work on childrearing unfortunately also had quite an impact in their day. His *Thoughts on Education,* published in 1690, convinced moms in England and America to bathe their babies in freezing water, dress them in thin-soled shoes so that the water could leak in, quench their thirst with beer, and never, never feed them fruit or meat.

Claudius I of Rome choked to death on a feather brandished by his physician. The doctor was using it to tickle the emperor's throat to try to induce vomiting. True, Claudius might have died anyway— his wife had been serving him poisonous mushrooms.

$5,000 is the amount Drs. Wilhelm Loeser and Harold B. Cassidy charged gangster John Dillinger to alter his facial features and remove his fingerprints. But perhaps Dillinger should have found another team. First of all, they managed to stop his heart with an overdose of ether, barely getting him resuscitated again. Second, the gangster's facial features were still recognizable enough for lawmen. The FBI caught up with him outside a theater in Chicago twenty-six days after he emerged from his bandages. They shot him dead.

In the 1920s, you could buy a chocolate candy bar called the Rejuvinator. It was laced with radium, the idea being that it would make you stronger. Not true. People knew that radioactivity could have near-magical properties in burning away certain cancers. However, they didn't know the dangers. Radium was mixed in with paint and put on walls and watch hands to make them glow in the dark. It was added to face cream, hair tonics, and toothbrushes. It wasn't until a decade later when an inordinate number of watch painters started dying of leukemia that it became clear how dangerous radioactivity could be.

Eight people were convicted of conspiracy in the assassination of Abraham Lincoln. One of them was Dr. Samuel Mudd, a physician who set John Wilkes Booth's broken leg and harbored him for twelve hours when Booth was a fugitive. Some historians believe Mudd was an innocent caregiver who didn't recognize Booth;

others point out that Booth had met with him in a hotel room at least once and sent liquor to him two weeks before the assassination. Dr. Mudd escaped the death penalty by one vote. While in prison, he distinguished himself during a yellow fever epidemic and was pardoned after four years of imprisonment. He resumed his practice.

In the early twentieth century, the Sears Roebuck catalog offered a wide range of the patent medicines and dubious medical devices of the day. One of them was "the anti-cancer cigar holder" with the claim that it guaranteed "a tongue burnt by properly smoking" to prevent tumors.

seven

Doctoring for Dollars

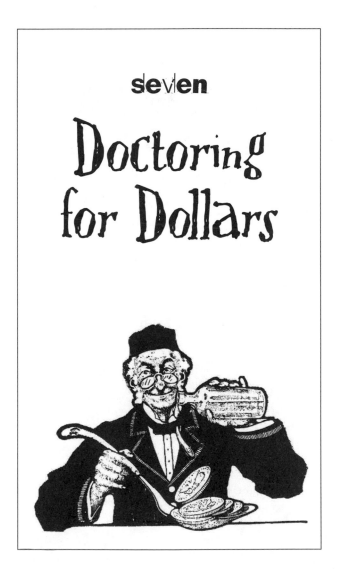

*"*inancial ruin from medical bills is almost exclusively an American disease."
—*Roul Turley, writer*

According to *The Jobs Rated Almanac*, 8 out of 10 of the best-paying professional careers are in the realm of medicine. The top ten are:

1. Surgeon
2. Orthodontist
3. Dentist
4. Psychiatrist
5. General practice physician
6. Podiatrist
7. Attorney
8. Financial planner
9. Osteopath
10. Optometrist

The average physician makes more than $165,000 every year.

Can't decide what specialty to go into? The lowest average starting salary in the medical profession is for oral and maxillo-facial surgeons. Consider a career in cardiovascular surgery: Those guys start out on average making about $208,000 a year—more than any other specialized medical field.

Of course, a dollar was a day's pay back then, but still. . . . Oswego, New York, medical records show that a typical patient in 1816 paid $1.25 to have a baby and 25¢ to have a tooth pulled.

How much did a doctor's house call cost a patient? The fee schedule fixed by the Clinton County Medical Society in upstate New York in the early 1800s was 25¢ for a day visit and 38¢ for a night visit, plus a fee of 20¢ per mile ridden.

The American Medical Association had a problem in the late 1940s: President Truman was proposing a nationwide health plan that the doctors' group was afraid might cut into its members' income. The AMA hired a PR firm that invented a new term that was deliberately designed to sound sinister and un-American: "socialized medicine." During those jittery anti-communist days, the name stuck and successfully sank Truman's program. In the 1960s, the "socialized medicine" phrase was dusted off by the medical industry to fight Kennedy's Medicare plan and Clinton's universal health plan, and any other time when plans emerged to extend basic health coverage to more of America's citizens.

In 2000, American prescription drug companies made $27 billion in profits. They spent $9.1 billion on advertising and free samples . . . and a mere $264 million on research and development.

Thanks to the economy of scale in its government health plan, the cost of prescription drugs in Canada is 61 percent cheaper than in the United States.

You think medicine is expensive today? In medieval Europe, alchemists mixed gold into drinks to comfort arthritis.

In ancient China, doctors were paid when their patients stayed well. The doctors paid the patients if the patient got sick. The idea was that the doctor's job was to keep the patient well.

In a similar scheme, in fifth-century France and Spain, the Visigoth rulers required doctors to leave a cash deposit with the family of each patient. If the patient died, the doctor forfeited his deposit and could not collect his bill.

The secret of success is repeat business: At the end of 6 out of 10 doctor visits, the patient is scheduled for another appointment.

"A hospital should also have a recovery room adjoining the cashier's office."
— *Francis O'Walsh, cultural commentator*

The first medical malpractice lawsuit on record—a plaintiff alleging that an inept physician maimed his hand—took place nearly 650 years ago in England.

New York has more malpractice suits filed against physicians than any other state.

If you sell your body to a medical institute, can you buy it back before you die? That was the question before a Swedish court in 1910. A financially desperate man had signed a contract with Stockholm's Caroline Institute promising to deliver his body after his death in exchange for money now. A few years later he came into some money and wanted to buy back rights to his body, but the school refused to sell them. After some deliberation, the court backed the school's right to do so . . . and furthermore, that the man had to pay the school damages for having two teeth extracted without permission.

"When I had my operation, the doctor
gave me a local anesthetic. I couldn't afford the imported kind."
—The 1960s TV variety show Laugh-In

It's estimated that $25 billion a year is lost
in U.S. productivity due to the common
headache.

How much is your human body worth?
The erroneous popular answer, breaking it
down to its basic elements, is usually something like $2.98. However, if you marketed
your individual body parts intelligently, di-
viding them into organs and complex
chemicals, your body is worth more than
$170,000 (and maybe more if auctioned
on eBay).

Actually, we were just kidding about eBay. The online auction site stopped all trading in human body parts after a man offered one of his kidneys in 1999. Bids had gotten up to $5.7 million when eBay stopped the auction.

Paging Doc Martens, Dr. Pepper, and Dr. Scholl

There really was a Dr. Pepper. Wade Morrison, the guy who invented the soft drink, once worked for a pharmacist in Virginia whose name was Kenneth Pepper.

Although it sounds like a made-up name, perhaps a combination of "shoe" with "sole," Dr. Scholl really was a doctor. In the late nineteenth century, William ("Billy") Scholl left his farm in LaPorte, Indiana, to become a shoemaker in Chicago. He noticed how much abuse the average foot took and decided to become a podiatrist. As part of his medical work, he began making arch supports and other foot aids, and thus his name lives on.

Graham crackers and graham flour are named in honor of Dr. Sylvester Graham, a fiery nutritionist in the 1830s and '40s. In a time when these were considered radical ideas, Graham advocated taking baths, brushing teeth, eating whole grains and vegetables, exercising, family planning, and laughing at the dinner table to aid digestion.

Perhaps you suspected as much, but kid's author Dr. Seuss was not really a doctor. As a student Theodore Geisel was caught with gin in his Dartmouth dorm room, and as punishment Geisel was forced to resign as editor from the school's humor rag. Instead, he used his middle name "Seuss" and kept at it. Years later, he added the "Dr." to sound more "scientific," he claims.

It became a semi-legitimate title in 1957 when his alma mater awarded Geisel an honorary doctorate.

You know Doc Martens' shoes: Was there really a Dr. Martens? Well . . . sort of. Dr. Klaus Maertens was a podiatrist who first designed orthopedic shoes for older women. After he expanded his line to include other ages and men in the late 1940s, a British shoe company—memories of World War II still fresh in memory—began selling Maertens' shoes with an Anglicized trade name.

Johnson & Johnson was the first company to offer sterile dressings to the medical community, but none of the brothers were doctors. The company should have, by right, been called Johnson, Johnson & Johnson, because it was founded by *three* brothers: Robert, James, and Edward. Siblings being what they are, Edward soon left the company and started the pharmaceutical/baby formula company Mead Johnson, using his middle and last name.

Dr. Harvey Kellogg was a real doctor who founded the Kellogg's cereal company with his brother William. Their first product, Kellogg's Corn Flakes, was designed to reduce sexual urges, which Dr. Kellogg believed was a good idea.

nine

Hospitals in General

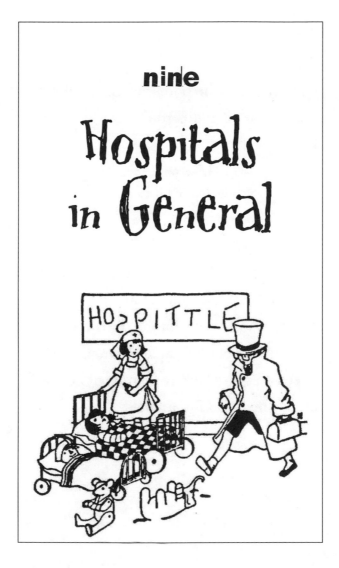

"Think of the money in hospitals. Do you know the mark-up on oxygen alone? Fantastic! And the poor customers, there's nothing they can do. You've got 'em flat on their backs!"

—*TV character Thalia Menninger,*
The Many Loves of Dobie Gillis

Hospitals date back to at least 437 B.C.E. , when one was established in Ceylon. A memorial in India from the third century B.C. honors King Priyadarschin, who "erected everywhere two kinds of hospitals, for men and for animals."

We suspect that the al-Mansur Hospital was not run by an HMO. This Cairo institution opened in 1284 and featured spacious wards cooled by fountains and entertained by musicians, storytellers, and fifty readers of the Koran. When discharged, patients were given pocket money so that they could afford to take some time off from work.

Unfortunately, during the same Middle Ages, European hospitals were squalid, fetid, deadly places. To counteract the overpowering stench, attendants would press vinegar-soaked sponges over their faces. Death rates for all patients, regardless of affliction, were in the 20 percent range. To deal with the problem, hospitals in some areas started requiring a burial deposit for all incoming patients.

"A trip to the hospital is always a descent in to the macabre. I have never trusted a place with shiny floors."

—*Terry Tempest Williams,*
naturalist and writer

The term "bedlam" comes from a lower-class pronunciation of London's Bethlehem Hospital, which was an insane asylum. "Treatment" within the bedlam at Bethlehem Hospital was primitive and brutal in those pre-Freudian days. One regimen, designed to prevent violence, was the flogging of selected inmates at certain stages of the moon.

Yes, he created America's first fire brigade, postal system, and anti-slavery organization, but did you know that Benjamin Franklin also helped establish America's first hospital? The Pennsylvania Hospital was founded in 1751 in Philadelphia, Pennsylvania.

The second U.S. hospital opened shortly afterward in New York City. Both made it their firm policy for "moral" reasons not to treat unwed mothers or patients with sexually transmitted diseases.

"Hospitals, like airports and supermarkets, only pretend to be open nights and weekends."

—*Molly Haskell, film critic*

"Looking out of a hospital window is different from looking out of any other. Somehow you do not see outside."

—Carol Matthau, Walter's wife

Mr. and Ms. David Harkness of Iowa were informed in 1993 that the hospital where they both worked had a policy against employing people married to each other. The otherwise happily wed couple traveled to Tijuana, Mexico, got a quick divorce, and continued to live and work together.

A survey taken a few years ago asked 10,000 U. S. nurses if they'd willingly choose to be patients in their own hospitals. Thirty-eight percent said, "No way."

According to the Centers for Disease Control and Prevention, 2 million patients in the United States develop a hospital-acquired infection each year, and 90,000 die as a result of those infections.

The rate at which patients pick up an infection while being treated in a U.S. hospital has increased 36 percent in the twenty years between 1978 and 1998.

"It's like a convent, the hospital. You leave the world behind and take vows of poverty, chastity, and obedience."

—*Carolyn Wheat, writer*

"In hospitals there is not time off for good behavior."

—*Josephine Tey, mystery writer*

To choose the healthiest location for a hospital in ninth-century Baghdad, doctors hung pieces of meat at each possible site. The location where the meat last turned rotten was the one they chose.

In 1929, Justin Ford Kimball, an official at Baylor University in Dallas, introduced a hospitalization plan for schoolteachers. Others imitated it; a Minnesota plan adopted a blue cross design modeled after the Red Cross. In 1939, the American Hospital Association trademarked the Blue

Cross name and symbol for plans that met its guidelines. The cost of Kimball's plan was a good deal. He guaranteed up to twenty-one days of hospital care . . . for $6 a year.

What's the difference between Blue Cross and Blue Shield? While Blue Cross was set up to cover hospital costs, Blue Shield covered the doctors' fees. The two groups merged in 1982, except in California where they remain separate companies.

"Hospitals are only an intermediate stage of civilization."

— *Florence Nightingale,*
nursing pioneer

Adding up all U.S. hospitals (general, psychiatric, chronic, etc.), you get a total of about 6,500.

The Irish Sweepstakes, for a while the only government-sponsored lottery in the world, was started in 1930 to benefit Irish hospitals. The Irish sold tickets worldwide, introducing many Canadians and Americans to the concept of sweepstakes.

Jimmy Carter was the first American president to have been born in a hospital.

Long before he wrote *One Flew over the Cuckoo's Nest,* Ken Kesey worked as an attendant in a mental hospital.

John Kennedy, Lee Harvey Oswald, and Jack Ruby all died in the same hospital: Parkland Hospital in Dallas.

ten

Just Say No

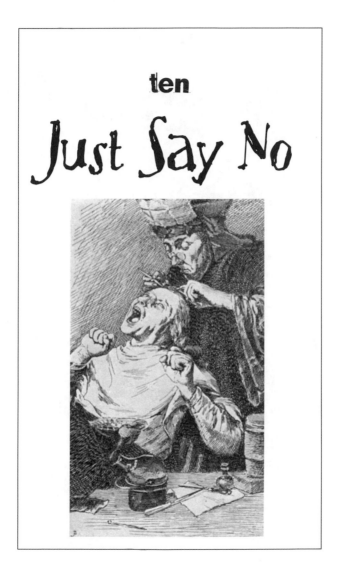

"He's the best physician who knows the worthlessness of most medicines."

—*Benjamin Franklin*

Calling Dr. Starbucks! In eighteenth-century England and France, doctors prescribed coffee for a variety of illnesses, from sore throats to smallpox.

Interns Take Note: It is possible to get a lethal dose of caffeine. Ten grams can kill the average human. That's the equivalent of about 100 cups of coffee over four hours (or, if drinking Starbucks, three or four cups).

A century ago, the laws in Hartford, Connecticut, forbade anyone from buying chewing tobacco without a permit from a doctor.

Karl Gerhardt discovered aspirin in 1853, but it took another half-century before doctors started routinely prescribing it to their patients.

Not that long ago, cobra venom was experimentally prescribed to relieve the pain of arthritis. It worked well for many people, but its serious side effects prevented it from being adopted widely. However, extracts of cobra venom continue to be investigated for possible use today, including for the treatment of AIDS.

In modern times, the venom of rattlers and other poisonous snakes has been used as painkillers (for arthritis, cancer, and leprosy), antispasmodics (for epilepsy and asthma), and blood coagulants (for hemophilia, tonsillectomies, and bleeding gums).

Capsaicin is the compound that makes chili peppers hot. Researchers rubbed it on the noses of people with headaches and found that 75 percent reported relief from pain . . . the headache pain, anyway.

Quaaludes were originally developed to fight malaria.

Thank a druggist's defective pill machine for the hole in Life Savers. When candy maker Clarence Crane decided to expand into mints, he jobbed the manufacturing out. "Unfortunately," the pill-pusher apologized, "the machine keeps punching a hole into the center of each one." Don't fix it, said Crane, keep it the way it is—they look like little life preservers. He built a campaign around saving yourself from "that stormy breath," and the rest is candy history.

Pharmacists have not always had the complete trust of the authorities. In fact, one of the earliest written references to drug stores was a decree by Frederick II of the Holy Roman Empire in 1240 that fixed the prices of drugs and forbade pharmacists from entering into secret financial agreements with doctors. The city of Dijon, France, in the fifteenth century prohibited pharmacists from being beneficiaries of their clients' wills. And in the sixteenth century, the French government required that druggists swear not to slander their teachers or masters nor "examine women privately, unless by great necessity."

The first modern tranquilizer was derived from the root of the Indian plant *Rauwolfia serpentina*. The plant had been used by Hindu physicians as early as the fourth century C.E., but Western medicine didn't discover it until the 1940s.

Thanks to opium's widespread use as a painkiller, more than 100,000 soldiers came out of the Civil War addicted to it.

Poisons used by South American natives on their arrow tips have been found to have medical applications and are used in Western medicine. One, a poison called curare, is used to relax patients' abdominal muscles during surgery. (It kills birds and animals by relaxing them so much that they can't breathe.) Another poison used on South American arrow tips is ouabain. It's very similar in make-up to the Western medicinal drug digitalis, which is used to treat congestive heart failure and congenital heart defects.

"'The pen is mightier than the sword!'— the case for prescriptions rather than surgery."

—*Marvin Kitman,*
TV critic and columnist

Inca surgeons used coca during operations long before the anaesthetic properties of cocaine were discovered in Europe. Here's the irony, though—they didn't use it on patients, they used it on *themselves* to keep their alertness level high while operating.

eleven

Medicine by the Numbers

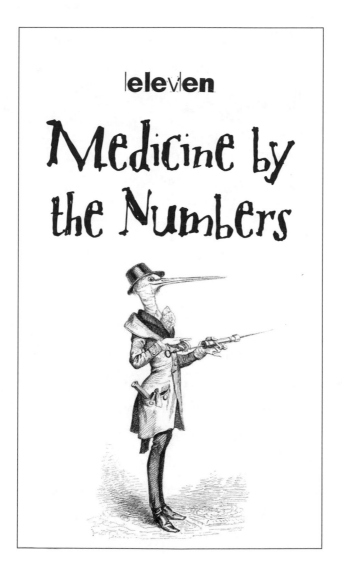

120: The number of toilet seat–related injuries American hospitals treat in an average day.

15,000: The number of Americans in comas.

6 million: The number of American knees treated by orthopedic surgeons each year.

18,000: The number of eyeballs lost to disease or injury last year. Good artificial eyes are indistinguishable from the real thing, but they don't come cheap—from $1,700 to $2,500 for a custom-made replica, usually covered by medical plans. But don't call them "glass eyes"; nowadays, they're made from unbreakable plastic.

60,000 miles: How long your circulatory system would be if laid out in a straight line—enough to circle the globe two and a half times.

The height of a three-story building: The length of your alimentary canal from mouth to anus if you straightened it out.

1.5 gallons: The amount of blood that an average man has; the average woman has .875 gallons.

13 tons: The amount of gold used each year by American dentists for fillings, crowns, inlays, and dentures.

9 million: The number of new cases of sexually transmitted diseases in the United States every year.

120 years: The legends about Methusulah notwithstanding, in all of recorded history the maximum human life span.

More than half: The number of all school-aged kids who now have no cavities in their teeth. This compares to only 26 percent in the early 1970s.

690,000: The number of licensed physicians in the United States and its colonies, according to the American Medical Association.

50: The number of patients, at last count, for which a single transplant donor can provide parts—organs, tissue, bone, and so on.

3 out of 4 Americans: How many will report foot problems of some sort at some time in their lives.

40,000 units of blood: The number used each day in the United States. That's about 5,000 gallons. Heart surgery can require only about 6 units of blood; a car crash victim may need 50.

20 minutes: The average wait in a doctor's office waiting room, according to the American Medical Association.

1/100th of an inch: The thickness of skin in a typical skin graft.

12,000: The number of surgeons in the United States who perform transgender operations.

21,655: The number of organs transplanted in 1999. Most of those—12,488—were kidney transplants. Another 48,395 patients are currently waiting for a healthy kidney.

8.4: The percentage of kidney dialysis patients who will live beyond the ten-year mark. However, following a kidney transplant, at least 57 percent have a chance of living more than ten years.

34,439: The number of doctors who volunteered to take part in a statistical study in 1951. Their lives, deaths, and sicknesses over the following years helped drive a coffin nail into the denial of what was long suspected: that smoking is a killer.

13 million: The number of adults who suffer from incontinence. At least $26.3 billion a year is spent on treating this condition in people aged sixty-five or older.

twelve

Bedside Manners

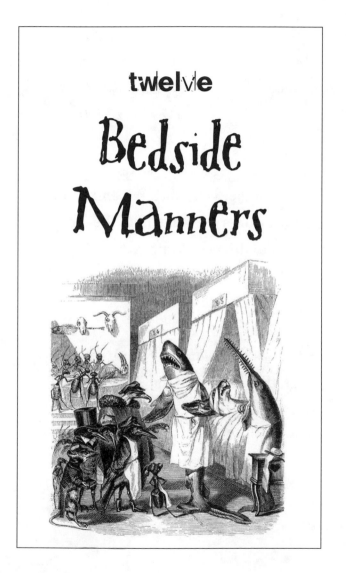

"Your patient has no more right to all the truth you know than he has to all the medicine in your bag."

—*Dr. Oliver Wendell Holmes*

"In medicine, as in statecraft and propaganda, words are sometimes the most powerful drugs we can use."

—*Dr. Sara Murray Jordan, medical author*

"One has a greater sense of intellectual degradation after an interview with a doctor than from any other human experience."

—*Alice James, diarist (1848–1892),
who incidentally was sister of
Henry and William James*

"The ultimate indignity is to be given a bedpan by a stranger who calls you by your first name."

—*Maggie Kuhn, founder of the Grey Panthers*

"The art of medicine consists in amusing the patient while nature cures the disease."

—*Voltaire French satirist (1694–1778)*

How do dentists keep their little mirrors from fogging up in your mouth? Maybe you didn't notice that they warm it up to body temperature against the inside of your cheek.

"My doctor gave me two weeks to live. I hope they're in August."

—*Rita Rudner,*
comedian

"To array a man's will against his sickness is the supreme art of medicine."

—*Henry Ward Beecher*

The language of medical workers has confused lay people through history. In 1699, poet Samuel Garth wrote:

The patient's ears remorselessly he assails—
Murders with jargon where his medicine
fails.

"**W**hen I told my doctor I couldn't afford an operation, he offered to touch up my x-rays."

—Henny Youngman,
comedian

"**I** quit therapy because my analyst was trying to help me behind my back."

—Richard Lewis,
comedian

"**S**how me a sane man and I will cure him for you."

—Dr. Carl Jung

"He is the best physician who is the most ingenious inspirer of hope."

—*Samuel Taylor Coleridge*

"Whoever is spared personal pain must feel himself called to help in diminishing the pain of others."

—*Dr. Albert Schweitzer*

"Care more for the individual patient than for the special features of the disease."

—*Sir William Osler,*
Canadian medical pioneer (1849–1919)

"One of the first duties of the physician is to educate the masses not to take medicine."

—*Sir William Osler*

In ancient China, it was considered inde-
cent for doctors to examine the bodies of
their female patients, or even to ask too
many probing personal questions. This
made diagnosis difficult, but not impossible. To work around the problem, doctors
gave their patients a small doll of a naked
woman and had them mark the parts that
were giving them trouble, and then made a
diagnosis based on that.

"Let the surgeon take care to regulate the
whole regimen of the patient's life for joy
and happiness, allowing his relatives and
special friends to cheer him, and by having some one tell him jokes. The surgeon
must forbid anger, hatred and sadness in

the patient and remind him that the body grows fat from joy and thin from sadness."

—*Henri de Mondeville,*
French professor of surgery (1260–1320)

In the fourteenth century, French physician Henri de Mondeville stressed the need for a good bedside manner in patient recovery. Like a Middle Ages Patch Adams, he used humor and violin music. He wasn't above lying to patients if he thought it would do a patient some good, suggesting that surgeons use "false letters about the deaths of his enemies, or—if he is a spiritual man—by telling him that he has been made a bishop."

"It is more important to know what sort of person has a disease than to know what sort of disease a person has."

—*Hippocrates (circa 460–380 B.C.E.)*

"One finger in the throat and one in the rectum makes a good diagnostician."

—*Dr. William Osler*

"To promote good health, we must study disease."

—*Plutarch (46–120 C.E.)*

"Wherever the art of medicine is loved, there also is a love of humanity."

—*Hippocrates*

"The true physician does not preach repentance; he offers absolution."

—H. L. Mencken,
satirist

"To be a doctor is to be an intermediary between man and God."

—Felix Marti-Ibanez,
author

"Losing your patients is not a virtue."

—Edward Zorn, humorist

thirteen

Alternative Medicine

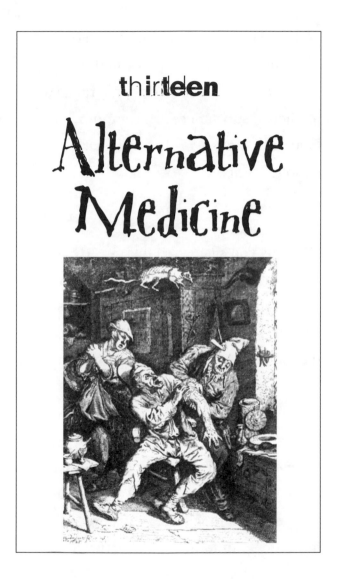

The first known drugstore opened for business in A.D. 754. Located in downtown Baghdad, it offered a wide range of medicinal substances like camphor, cloves, tamarind, sandalwood, marijuana, and alcoholic spirits.

Perhaps you suspected this already, but the inventor of acupuncture wasn't a doctor. The practice is credited to the Chinese Emperor Shen Nung in 2700 B.C.E., or thereabouts, to treat problems with the heart, circulation, and pulse.

Trepanning—drilling a hole in the skull— is the most ancient form of surgery, dating from the Neolithic Age. It was prescribed for patients suffering from fractured skulls, convulsions, epilepsy, insanity, and headaches. Trepanning is still used today to reduce pressure in the skull.

Lady-killer Henry VIII believed that he'd invented a cure for syphilis: a paste of powdered pearls and guaiacum resin from the New World that he marketed as "The King's Majesty's Own Plaster."

A Good Idea at the Time: The *pil perpetuae,* a laxative product sold in seventeenth-century Europe. It consisted of a pellet of the element antimony. Although it was expensive, it had a thrifty selling point: As its name suggests, the *pil perpetuae* was long-lasting—when you swallowed it, it did its work and passed through your body pretty much unchanged. You and your loved ones could retrieve it, wash it off, and use it over and over again.

In A.D. 43, a Roman doctor first used electricity to fight pain, using an electricity-generating fish to provide the juice. Unfortunately, the treatment had some side effects in that an occasional patient was electrocuted.

Black pepper was once thought to have many medicinal properties. In 400 B.C., Hippocrates recommended it for women's reproductive complaints, and a century later Theophrastus prescribed it as an antidote for hemlock poisoning.

A-Choo!

During plague periods, the Romans started the custom of saying "Jupiter bless you" when people sneezed. Pope Gregory the Great followed suit during a plague in the sixth century, ushering in the European custom of saying "God bless you" when someone sneezes.

Among seventeenth-century European doctors, sneezing was considered a sign that a patient was shedding the ill humors that were bringing on sickness. A patient who sneezed three times would be discharged from a hospital as someone who was clearly on the road to recovery.

Hindus also saw sneezing as a good sign. It meant that an evil spirit was being released. It was then the responsibility of a sneezer to quickly issue a blessing and give a snap of the fingers to keep the demon from taking up residence in an onlooker.

Hippocrates' favorite toothpaste was made by burning three mice and a hare's head to extract tricalcium phosphate. Pliny the Elder liked burnt eggshells. George Washington's toothpaste (before and after losing his teeth) was chalk. Other toothpastes used through time included rust, wine vinegar, pumice, powdered crab eyes, bat excrement, and human urine.

State-of-the-art medicine in prehistoric times was designed to keep alien demon spirits from infecting the body. Preventive medicine included magic, charms, incantations, and talismans. If, despite preventive measures, demons entered a patient's body, prehistoric medical personnel drove them out by inducing violent vomiting. If that didn't work, making the body inhospitable to the spirit was the next step, and so caregivers would provide a regimen of beating, torturing, and starving. In especially resistant demons, a hole drilled into the head was prescribed to encourage the demon to escape.

"Like cures like" was an old medical concept. Early doctors noticed that shelled walnuts look like a tiny brain, and so prescribed walnuts for brain diseases.

In Germany of old, pediatric specialists suggested soothing a teething baby's gums by rubbing them with sheep brains.

Ancient Egyptians believed that the heart was the center of intelligence and emotions. The brain was considered an insignificant mass of tissue. In preparing the dead for their trip to the next world, mummifiers carefully preserved the other organs but pulled the brain out in pieces through the nose and discarded it.

Forget the heart or the brain—smart guy Aristotle insisted that the liver was the seat of all human emotions.

True, Hippocrates' oath wasn't half-bad (although there's still some controversy as to whether he actually wrote it). However, the ancient was as bound as anybody by the ignorance of his place and time. For example, he believed that veins carried air and that illness came from vapors emanating from undigested food in the bowels.

In the 1100s, doctors in Europe and Asia began grinding mummies into a powder for use as a tea or poultice for its supposed health benefits. It was prescribed for nausea, epilepsy, migraines, coughs, bruises, fractures, paralysis, and as an antidote for poisoning. Not everybody thought the powder itself was good enough, however; French doctors insisted that a better medicine came from boiling the mummies and skimming off the mummy oil that rose to the top.

Supplies of pharmaceutical-grade mummy powder were plentiful and cheap—a Scot noted that the going rate in the 1800s was about 8 shillings for a pound. Besides the alleged health benefits, artists added it to their paints, figuring the magic in the mummies would keep the colors from fading over time.

The use of mummy powder declined in the seventeenth century, as the medical world eventually agreed with French surgeon Ambrose Peré, who wrote that "not only does this wretched drug do no good, but it causes great pain to the stomach, gives foul-smelling breath, and brings on serious vomiting." We can imagine.

Besides leeches and bloodletting, there were other colorful cures from the dark ages of medicine. Here are some of the cures that you may not get from your personal caregiver:

"To draw out the venom of a plague sore, cut a live pigeon in two and apply one of the halves."

"For satyriasis [overactive male libido] leape into a great fessel of cold water or put nettles in the codpiece."

"For gout, swallow scrapings from a hanged man's skull."

"**O**il of swallows" was a popular cure in the Middle Ages. Here's the process of making it, as explained by a pharmacist's handbook:

> Take young swallows of their nest, by number twelve, rosemary tips, bay leaves, of each a handful; cut off the long feathers of the swallows, wings and tails, put them into a stone mortar and lay the herbs upon them and beat them all to pieces, guts, feathers, bones and all.

The medical schools of the Middle Ages continued to teach what had been taught for centuries: that disease was caused by the imbalance of the "four humors": blood, phlegm, yellow bile, and black bile; and that health was affected by the "five inertia": stars, food, mind, divine purpose, and poisons. The faculty of the finest medical schools in Europe debated weighty issues like which of the precious crystals had the greatest therapeutic value.

Although tomatoes were once considered poisonous, in the 1830s ketchup achieved some popularity as a patent medicine: "Dr. Miles's Compound Extract of Tomato."

For centuries in Europe the stings of bees have been used to successfully relieve arthritis, rheumatism, gout, and other painful joint conditions. Modern-day practitioners call it "apitherapy" and keep hives of bees around for that very purpose.

Marijuana and a strong wine—the combination was the first known general anesthesia used in surgery. Chinese physician Hua T'a used it while operating during the second century A.D.

In the seventeenth century, the prescribed regimen for the plague was to hold a succession of live chickens next to your plague carbuncles in the hope that the fowl would "draw out the poisons." Did it work? No better than anything else, but it was standard treatment for much of the century.

In Europe during the sixteenth through eighteenth centuries, the color red was thought to be therapeutic in bringing down fevers, so patients wore red nightclothes and surrounded themselves with red objects.

The Flagellants appeared first in four-teenth-century Germany, whipping and beating each other into religious ecstasy. They believed that if they punished them-selves for the sins of humanity, God would stop the plagues that continually ravaged Europe at that time. He did . . . eventually.

The World Health Organization has listed more than 20,000 plants that are being used for therapeutic purposes in both medicinal and herbal remedies.

Sugar 'n' Spice 'n' Extra Years of Life: Here's another health theory not likely to survive its real-life trials. In 1743, Dr. John Cohausen wrote a book called *Hemippus Redivivus,* in which he claimed that people could live to 115 years of age by regularly inhaling the exhaled breath of little girls.

The jaws of ants are strong, and they continue to grip even after death. Since the tenth century B.C.E., health care professionals in tropical areas have used large ants as sutures. The wound was held shut, and one by one ants were held over the closed edges. When each ant bit, the caregiver decapitated it.

Cauterization with boiling oil or a red-hot iron was used for centuries to stop bleeding. Ow.

In ancient Greece, runners somehow got the impression that the spleen was a hindrance to their speed and endurance. Their doctors obligingly created a panoply of herbal concoctions made from horsetail reed, meant to shrink this vital organ.

While some physicians claimed to be able to shrink the spleen, Dr. Hippocrates claimed that he knew of a certain mushroom that, when burned near the body, made the spleen disappear altogether.

Are onions medicine? Folk wisdom would tell you they are. Here are some of the potential cures of this wonder drug:

Fever: Drink onion tea.

Headache: Rub an onion on your head.

Chest cold: Rub fried onions and turpentine on your chest.

In case you're suspicious of modern medicine, here are some more tidbits of folk wisdom. Try them in good health.

Rheumatism: Wear an eel skin around your waist.

Chicken pox: Lie on the floor and have someone chase a flock of chickens over you.

Freckles: Rub face with live frog.

Frostbite: Rub with a mix of milk and cow manure.

Here's a medicine that cures most ills: chocolate! Actually, the Aztecs believed it also had wondrous properties. They used it believing that it cures dysentery, acts as an aphrodisiac, and, in large quantities, helps you see the god Quetzalcoatl.

When surgeons in ancient Babylon were stymied by a case, they covered their patient with a thin layer of clay and watched to see where it hardened first. That was where they operated. The idea was that the sickest, most infected part of the body generated the most body heat.

In the 1300s, French soldiers carried spider webs in their first-aid kits. When packed into wounds, the webs stopped the bleeding.

What did hospitals use in surgery before anaesthetic to keep the patient still? "Holders down"—burly guys who pinned screaming patients to the operating table and kept them from writhing.

During the days of bloodletting as a "cure," the affluent would go to surgeons. Poor people would try to get the same "benefits" by wading in leech-filled ponds.

It's easy to laugh at outlandish folk medicines of the past, but consider this: In 2001, a mysterious ancient Chinese potion made of ground rock and toad venom was investigated as a promising experimental cancer treatment at Sloane-Kettering Hospital in New York. Scientists had no idea why, but the arsenic trioxide in the potion appeared to cure a particularly devastating kind of leukemia.

fourteen

Medical Warnings

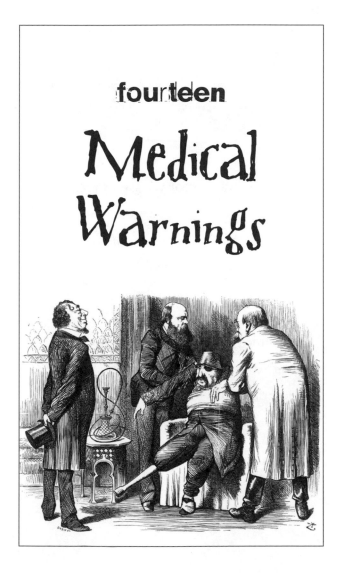

"Never play cards with a man called Doc."

—*Nelson Algren, American author (1909–1981)*

"Never go to a doctor whose office plants have died."

—*Erma Bombeck, humorist (1927–1996)*

"I was going to have cosmetic surgery until I noticed that the doctor's office was full of portraits by Picasso."

—*Rita Rudner, comedian*

"By medicine life may be prolonged, yet death will seize the doctor too."

—*William Shakespeare*

"There are more old drunkards than old doctors."

—*Benjamin Franklin*

The National Health Foundation once recommended that after suffering a cold you should wait at least six days before kissing someone.

Here's an irony: Health warnings may have caused an explosive increase in cigarette smoking. In 1910, public health officials successfully campaigned against chewing tobacco, warning that the resulting sputum could spread tuberculosis and other diseases, so many tobacco users switched to smoking. As ashtrays replaced cuspidors, lung cancer began edging out tuberculosis as the major lung disease.

Anti-tobacco forces struggled to catch up with this new development. In 1914, they circulated a letter from Thomas A. Edison, himself addicted to cigars. He wrote that unlike cigar smoke, the smoke from a paper-wrapped cigarette "has a violent action in the nerve centers, producing degeneration of the cells of the brain, which is quite rapid among boys. Unlike most narcotics, this degeneration is permanent and uncontrollable. I employ no person who smokes cigarettes." Buttressed by such authoritative though erroneous statements from respected public figures, the anti-cigarette campaigns successfully lobbied lawmakers. By 1921—the year after alcohol prohibition—fourteen states had enacted cigarette prohibition, and anti-cigarette bills were under consideration in twenty-eight state legislatures. Not surprisingly, considering the addictiveness of tobacco, people went right on smoking despite the laws. Finally, the last of the statewide cigarette prohibition laws was repealed in 1927.

"The English disease" was the name first given by the rest of Europe to bronchitis and emphysema. Between cigarette smoking and the polluted "fog" of its major cities, England got more than its share of cases during the Industrial Revolution.

In 1978, there was a sudden 60 percent drop in the number of organs donated for transplant. What was causing it, nervous transplant specialists asked? It didn't take long to figure out an unsettling coincidence at the local multiplex: Coma, a scary movie about murdering hospital patients for their organs, was playing to large crowds of potential donors. . . .

"**A** doctor's reputation is made by the number of eminent men who die under his care."

—*George Bernard Shaw*

A feature of Chinese medicine in ancient times acted as a sort of Consumer's Report. If a patient died, the grieving family hung a special lantern outside his doctor's house. The effect was that doctors with a lot of fatalities started losing business.

fifteen

Life Outside Medicine

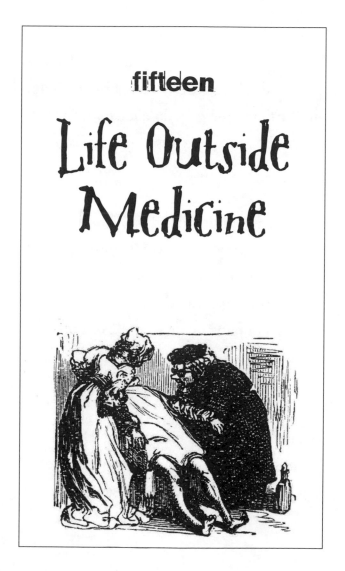

Sir T. O. Gimlette, a British naval surgeon, developed the Gimlet in 1890 as a healthful beverage. "Healthful"? Hmm, one part gin, one part lime juice . . . well, maybe the lime juice might prevent scurvy.

Who invented the bland baby food, Pablum? Three doctors at Toronto's Hospital for Sick Children, who were trying to prevent the crippling disease of rickets. Pablum contains no eggs, milk, or nuts but plenty of vitamin D.

Dr. Livingstone, I Presume? Dr. David Livingstone, the famous African explorer, was first a physician from Glasgow.

Hubert Humphrey kept his pharmacist license to fall back on in case his thirty-one-year political career didn't pan out.

Pill-Pushing Pen Pushers: Famous writers who were also pharmacists include O. Henry (William Sydney Porter), Henrik Ibsen, Dante Alighieri, and Johann Wolfgang von Goethe.

Elementary, my dear Dr. Watson—Sir Arthur Conan Doyle was a medical doctor when he wasn't writing Sherlock Holmes stories. A professor at med school had been his inspiration for Sherlock Holmes. At the Royal Infirmary at Edinburgh, Doyle studied under surgeon Dr. Joseph Bell and was impressed with Bell's deductive reasoning.

For example, Bell would often deduce the birthplace, class, military service, career, and travels of a person merely by paying close attention to things like positions of calluses on the hands and the way the person talked and walked. The point Dr. Bell was trying to make was the importance of observing subtleties in medicine; however, the point that Doyle got was that a brilliant detective using the same methods could make for entertaining reading.

Master of plays and short stories, Anton Chekhov was also a medical doctor.

Before the American Revolutionary War, both patriot Benjamin Franklin and traitor Benedict Arnold had been pharmacists.

Pharmacists who were pioneers in other fields include Sir Isaac Newton, who had a shop in Woolsthorpe, England, before putting his mind toward physics, and voyager Amerigo Vespucci, the druggist from Florence, Italy, for whom America was named.

Dr. Kildare, the fictional medical professional of books, radio, and TV, was created by writer Max Brand, who was most famous for his cowboy stories.

In the roster of pop-culture medical doctors who don't reflect well on the profession, include the character of Dr. Henry Jekyll, created by Robert Lewis Stevenson. Jekyll's self-medication experiments turned him into the sociopathic Mr. Edward Hyde, with fatal side effects. After dreaming the story, Stevenson, despite suffering from tuberculosis, wrote the 60,000-word classic in a six-day, cocaine-fueled frenzy.

Another evil fictitious pop-culture medical doctor: Dr. Fu Manchu. This villain of book and screen had medical degrees from three universities: Heidelberg, Edinburgh, and the Sorbonne. He was schooled in all major languages (and many minor ones), as well as chemistry and botany. If only he had used that intelligence for good, like curing cancer, solving the diseases borne of poverty, or revamping America's health care system. . . .

Celebrated dentists? That list would have to include:

Dr. G. W. A. Bonwill: Perfected the modern safety pin.

Dr. William Lowell: Invented the modern wooden golf tee.

Dr. Thomas Welch: Originated Welch's grape juice.

Doc Holliday: Wounded with the Earp brothers at the OK Corral.

Paul Revere: While famous as a silversmith, did dental work on the side.

Dr. Pearl Zane Grey: Wrote western novels (dropping his title and first name for his literary works) between seeing patients.

The unluckiest moonlighting dentist has to be Mahlon Loomis, who invented wireless telegraphy thirty-five years before Marconi. Unfortunately, he lost his financial backers after a market crash in 1869 and had to abandon the project.

Maybe he was merely trying to drum up business, but it was a dentist named William F. Semple who first added sugar and flavorings to chicle to make chewing gum. This was in 1869.

Bestselling baby doc Dr. Benjamin Spock had one more claim to fame: He competed in the 1924 Olympics' rowing competition.

"World War I ambulance driver" doesn't seem like a promising item on a résumé. Yet a number of creative people filled the job, including Walt Disney, Ernest Hemingway, Dashiell Hammett, e. e. cummings, W. Somerset Maugham, John Dos Passos, and Archibald MacLeish.

sixteen

Women & Medicine

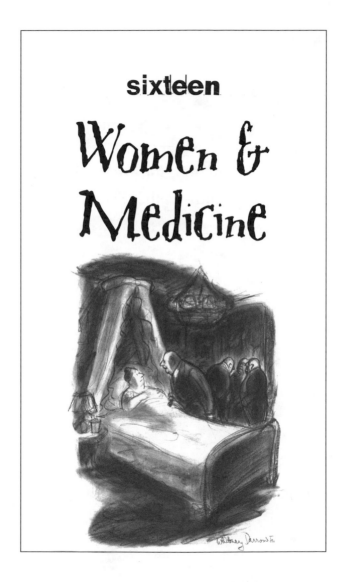

Remember this on Valentine's Day: Women reject heart transplants more often than men.

The first person hung for witchcraft during the seventeenth-century Salem, Massachusetts witch hunts was a midwife, Margaret Jones.

"I have so little sex appeal that my gynecologist calls me 'sir.'"

—*Joan Rivers*

"A male gynecologist is like an auto mechanic who has never owned a car."

—*Carry Snow, comedian*

"When a menstruating woman approaches, fermenting wine will be soured, seeds she touches become infertile, grass withers, garden plants shrivel, and fruit falls from the trees."

—*Gaius Secundus Pliny,*
Roman medical expert (A.D. 23–79)

In 1970, only 9 percent of medical students were female; by 2001, the figure had become 45 percent.

An analysis of appointment records indicates that women psychiatrists as a group see their patients more often than male psychiatrists.

Keeping Abreast

Early in the twentieth century a medical researcher wanted to quantify the range of "normal" in female breast size. He devised a measuring device consisting of a large, open-ended hypodermic plunger. When the plunger was pulled back, suction pulled the breast in where it could be visually measured.

In 1986, Australian doctors studying lactation wanted a more exact method of determining breast volume. Luckily, Western Australia has a large mining industry and its surveyors measure huge quantities of ore using a stereo camera in an airplane. "Stockpiles of ore viewed from an altitude

of about 1000 meters have similar charac-
teristics to a breast viewed from a distance
of about one meter," the doctors reported.
"This led to the concept of measuring the
volume of the breast stereoscopically." The
doctors recruited surveyors from a local
mining company who used their equip-
ment to measure the volume of volunteers'
breasts. "Unfortunately the breast was
smoother and had a more uniform color
than ore bodies, presenting problems for
the stereoscopic measurement technique,"
reported the doctors. "Nevertheless, it was
possible to calculate breast volume (albeit
in metric tons!)." Emboldened by this success, the doctors came up with a way to
miniaturize the process.

With early attempts at breast implants, surgeons tried using chunks of skin and fat, paraffin oil, carved ivory, and even little glass balls. Not surprisingly, they were failures—the implants migrated, were rejected by the body, or were absorbed into it.

1895 marked the first successful surgical breast augmentation. Killing two birds with one stone, a surgeon removed a fatty growth from a woman's leg and used it to fill a gap left from removing a benign tumor from her breast.

In a 1912 paper on hysteria, Sigmund Freud wrote that anxiety neurosis in women was often the result of their husbands depriving them of semen by practicing *coitus interruptus* or *coitus reservatus.*

According to patient statistics, as many as 30 percent of all women suffer from menstrual disorders and seek medical care for them.

Although abortion is one of the most common surgical procedures, by 1995, most medical schools had stopped providing training, and only 12 percent of ob/gyn residents were trained in the procedure. By the year 2001, only about 2,000 U.S. doctors provided the procedure, and most of them were in their fifties and sixties.

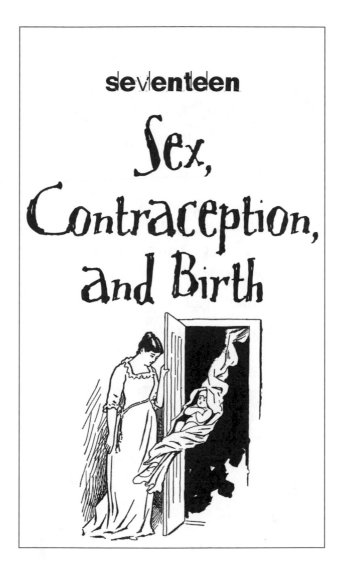

seventeen

Sex, Contraception, and Birth

Despite fears of heart patients, coronary thrombosis—blood clotting in the coronary arteries—is less likely to happen during sex than when resting, thanks to increased arterial blood flow.

I'm Coming, Lord! A medical journal in 1754 alleged that a man set out to commit suicide by sex. After having intercourse eighteen times in ten hours, he died. The effect on his partner (or partners) was not reported.

Anthropologists believe that it was only about 8,000 years ago that people caught on that men had something to do with starting pregnancy.

The earliest known recipe for countering conception was found on an Egyptian papyrus from about 4,000 years ago. It calls for a barrier made of lint coated with powdered acacia leaves. The slight acidity of the leaves might've actually been somewhat effective.

Working from the same approach, the famous lover Casanova advocated using a lemon half in the eighteenth century.

Other early female attempts at physical or chemical sperm barriers included mustard seeds, dried figs, beeswax, and crocodile droppings. On the male side, goat bladders, leather, linen, and large seed pods were all used.

For centuries, camel drivers inserted pebbles in the wombs of their camels before long trips to prevent them from becoming pregnant but didn't apparently consider that approach with their mates. Meanwhile, their wives tried a camel-related approach that probably didn't work: they collected and swallowed the froth from a camel's mouth.

What are the top two reasons that females aged from fifteen to twenty go to doctors?

1. Pregnancy
2. Acne

The "elephant man" was called that because it was standard medical wisdom at the time that his mother must've been scared at the zoo by an elephant.

Expectant mothers in the past were told to avoid animals at zoos, especially "ugly" animals like bears, giraffes, and apes. They were expected to surround themselves with lovely things and avoid ugly thoughts to avoid having an ugly baby. One hospital in the 1600s went so far as to ban ugly doctors from the maternity wards in the fear that the influence of their homeliness would create a generation of ugly babies.

Why obstetricians should vacation in February: The most popular month for giving birth is August, with 9.3 percent of all births, followed by October (9 percent).

"**G**iving birth is like trying to push a piano through a transom."

—Alice Roosevelt Longworth, socialite,
Teddy Roosevelt's daughter

How accurate is the obstetrician's estimated date of arrival? Not so good. Only about 1 baby in 40 arrives on the due date. Twice as many babies are born *after* the doctor's estimated date as are born before it.

Into the 1920s, babies in Finland were often delivered in saunas in the belief that the heat would fight infection and that the humid warm air would make transition from the womb to the world easier for baby.

"When I was born I was so surprised I didn't talk for a year and a half."

—*Gracie Allen,*
comedian (1906?–1964)

When Pablo Picasso was born, he wouldn't start breathing. Finally, his uncle, a doctor, blew cigar smoke into his mouth and nose. That did the trick.

When a newborn's lungs expand, about 20 ml of blood are sucked into its body from the placenta—making up much of the baby's total blood volume. That's a reason why the umbilical cord isn't cut until after the baby's first lusty cry.

Through the seventeenth century in Europe, midwives and doctors tied umbilical cords of boy babies as long as possible in the belief that a long cord would inspire their penises to grow longer.

"I never understood the fear of some parents about babies getting mixed up in the hospital. What difference does it make as long as you get a good one?"

—Heywood Brown, journalist

Standard medical procedure for premature babies before the twentieth century was to assume they would die. French pediatricians Pierre Budin and Martin Couney designed the first incubators for preemies in the 1890s, but they couldn't get investors or medical acceptance for the idea of using them. To garner both, they began to set up exhibits of "incubator babies" at World's Fairs and even amusement parks.

Dr. Couney's work in America included a very popular display at Coney Island that ran for forty years. Parents of the babies in the incubators paid nothing for their medical care; the costs of 24-hour care and wet nurses were paid for by the quarters of patrons who watched the babies through protective glass. More than 8,000 premature babies were saved by the sideshow exhibits. By the middle of the twentieth century, the results finally shamed obstetrical hospitals into investing in their own incubators.

Spring Up, Fall Out: Generally, children grow about twice as fast in the spring than in the fall and gain more weight in the fall than in the spring.

leighteen

What's in a Name?

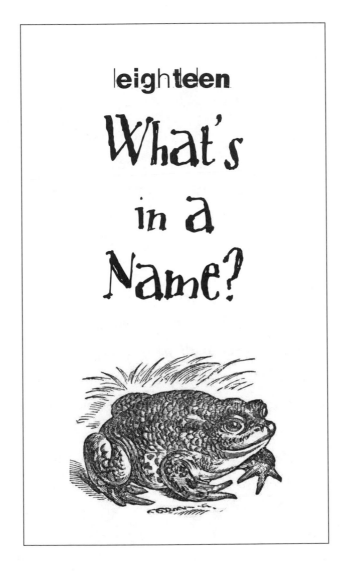

In medicalspeak, it's not a "black eye," it's a "bilateral periorbital hematoma."

Priapism—a prolonged and painful erection—is named after the Greek god Priapus, god of fertility and sexuality, who is usually depicted with an enormous penis.

Catgut has long been used in stitching up wounds, but have you ever wondered if catgut was ever made of—er, cat guts? The answer is no; it's made from sheep and pig intestines. So why is it called catgut? The most likely explanation is that it was a derivative of kit, the name for a small violin, for which the material used for its strings.

Why was rabies called "hydrophobia" in the old days? One of the strangest symptoms of the disease is this: The act of drinking water immediately induces violent throat spasms of the throat with choking, gagging, and a growing sense of panic. As the disease progresses, even the sight or sound of water triggers these reactions.

In the 1800s, *doctor* was used more indiscriminately than it is today. Druggists and undertakers were also addressed by that title.

In medicine shows, a "toad-eater" was an underling who'd pretend to eat poisonous toads so that the quack practitioner could demonstrate how his miracle patent medicine cured anything. It's where we got the word *toady*.

In Napoleon III's time, the French army decided that it was barbaric to leave wounded men on the battlefield until the end of the battle. So, they equipped a military stretcher with medical supplies and called it *le hospital ambulent*—"walking hospital" in French. From that we got the word *ambulance*.

English sailors were given limes to prevent scurvy on long ocean trips, which is how they got the nickname "limeys." (Although a colorful nickname never came from it, American sailors were given cranberries for the same reason.)

It's called a "vaccine" because Dr. Edward Jenner's first successful smallpox vaccine in 1796 was derived from cows—*vacca* in Latin.

Why are they called "vitamins"? It was partly a mistake. Casimir Funk, the American biochemist first named them "vitamines." He had rightly believed they were vital to life, so he began with *vita*. He also believed that they belonged to the *amine* chemical group. When the latter belief was proved wrong, he dropped the *e*.

Hired to help the French government distinguish feebleminded from normal children, psychologist Alfred Binet invented the IQ test. In analyzing the results, Binet labeled each child as "normal," "moron" (having the mental capability of a nine-year-old), "imbecile" (five-year-old), or "idiot" (two-year-old).

Mysophobia is the intense fear of picking up an infection.

The x in x-ray comes from the mathematical symbol for something unknown. Its discoverer, Dr. Wilhelm Roentgen, was a professor of mathematics and philosophy, not a physician.

"Half of 'analysis' is 'anal.'"

— *Marty Indik, humorist*

Salmonella is not named after the fish. It's named after the pathologist who discovered it, Dr. Daniel E. Salmon.

In the sixteenth century, Gabriel Fallopius discovered both the uterine oviduct, which now bears his name, and the eardrum, which doesn't. The fallopian tubes were named by somebody else in his honor, but Fallopius got in his own coinages as well. He gave names to the vagina, placenta, clitoris . . . and the ear canal.

Did a man named Guillotine invent the guillotine? No, it was a French physician named Dr. Antoine Louis. Why is the machine named "guillotine" then and not "louis"? Dr. Joseph Guillotin was a prominent Paris physician and was also a member of the French National Assembly. He spoke out about how inhumane execution by axe was—sometimes it took as many as half a dozen chops before the head was severed. The Assembly commissioned a search for a more humane method, and, to his later chagrin, the good doctor's name became attached to it. (Years later, the doctor's descendents, fed up with the burden of the family name, attempted to get the government to change the name of the execution device. When the government refused, the family gave up and changed its own name.)

Italian scientist Girolamo Fracastoro invented the name for syphilis. A poet as well as a physician, he wrote a poem called "Syphilis" about a shepherd infected with the disease. Syphilis was the shepherd's name, but eventually the affliction came to be known as "Syphilis' disease," and then just "syphilis." Before that, it was called *morbus gallicus* ("the disease of the French").

Oxygen, nitrous oxide, and nine other gases were first distilled by clergyman chemist Joseph Priestley using a technique he called "pneumatic chemistry." He certainly had a way with words—his original name for oxygen was "dephlogisticated air."

Morpheus was the Greek god of dreams and one of the sons of Hypnos, the god of sleep. He gave his name to morphine in 1805.

Influenza means "influence" in Italian. The illness was named that in 1743 because doctors believed its spread was under the influence of certain evil stars and constellations.

Ever wonder what that "R_x" symbol stands for on prescription forms? One theory proposes that it was was originally the astrological symbol for the planet Jupiter: ♃. In the Middle Ages, doctors believed that the planets and stars influenced health. Jupiter was supposed to be the most powerful in increasing the healing powers of medicines, so they may have figured that writing its name on medicines couldn't hurt.

Autopsy comes from the Greek words meaning "to see for yourself."

In 1638, Europeans discovered that the bark of a New World tree they called "cinchona" was useful in the treatment of malaria. The bark's active ingredient is quinine; the tree was named in honor of the Countess Chinchón, wife of the Spanish viceroy of Peru, whose fever was cured by it.

The name "aspirin" began as a brand name of the Bayer pharmaceutical company. It got its name like this: *a* from acetylsalicylic acid (its chemical name); *spir* from the original source of the compound, *Spiraea ulmaria,* the meadowsweet plant; and *in* because a lot of companies were ending their drug names with it in the late nineteenth century, and Bayer liked the sound of it.

Like "aspirin," the name "heroin" also began as a brand name of the Bayer pharmaceutical company. Bayer sold Heroin as an over-the-counter medicine. At the time, doctors believed that morphine addiction somehow occurred in the stomach and that an injectable opiate would solve that problem. The Heroin name came from *hero* because the company believed that it was a safe, nonaddictive substitute for morphine. Nowadays, the company advertisements for Heroin are prized as a macabre novelty by collectors.

Acknowledgments

The authors wish to warmly thank Conari editors Leslie Berriman, Pam Suwinsky, and Heather McArthur for their hard work in helping this book come together. Plus, a happy Hello to Elana, Eric, Jackson, and Georgia.

Selected References

Books

Anchor Bible Dictionary, ed. by David Noel Freedman. Doubleday & Company, 1992.

The Book of Answers: The New York Public Library Telephone Reference Service's Most Unusual and Entertaining Questions, by Barbara Berliner with Melinda Corey and George Ochoa. Fireside Books, 1990.

A Book of Legal Lists: The Best and Worst in American Law, by Bernard Schwartz. Oxford University Press, 1997.

The Compact Edition of the Oxford English Dictionary. Oxford University Press, 1985.

The Completely Amazing, Slightly Outrageous State Quarters Atlas and Album, by the editors of Klutz. Klutz, Inc., 2001.

Curious Punishments of Bygone Days, by Alice Morse Earle, 1896.

Encyclopaedia Britannica, ed. by the faculties of the University of Chicago. Benton Publishing, 1979.

Funny Laws, by Earle and Jim Harvey. Signet, 1982.

The Guinness Book of Records: 1999, by Guinness Publishing Ltd. Bantam Books, 1999.

Isaac Asimov's Book of Facts: 3,000 of the Most Interesting, Entertaining, Fascinating, Unbelieveable, Unusual and Fantastic Facts, ed. by Isaac Asimov.

Random House Value Publishing, Inc. edition, 1997.

The Juicy Parts: Things Your History Teacher Never Told You About the 20th Century's Most Famous People, by Jack Mingo. Perigee Books, 1996.

Jumbo Quiz Book. Helicon Publishing Ltd., 1996.

Just Curious, Jeeves, by Jack Mingo and Erin Barrett. Ask Jeeves, Inc., 2000.

Law 101: Everything You Need to Know about the American Legal System, by Jay M. Feinman. Oxford University Press, 2000.

Medical Curiosities: A Miscellany of Medical Oddities, Horrors and Humors, by Robert M. Youngson. Carroll & Graf, 1997.

News from the Fringe: True Stories of Weird People and Weirder Times, compiled by John J. Kohut and Roland Sweet. Plume Books, 1993.

The Oxford Dictionary of Quotations, Third Edition, by Book Club Associates. Oxford University Press, 1980.

Panati's Extraordinary Origins of Everyday Things, by Charles Panati. Harper & Row Publishing, 1987.

The People's Almanac Presents the Book of Lists, by David Wallechinsky and Amy Wallace. Little, Brown, 1993.

Peter's Quotations: Ideas for Our Time From Socrates to Yogi Berrs, Gems of Brevity, Wisdom, and Outrageous Wit, by Dr. Laurence J. Peter. William Morrow and Company, Inc., 1977.

Prime Time Proverbs: The Book of TV Quotes, by Jack
Mingo and John Javna. Harmony Books, 1989.

Stories Behind Everyday Things: Strange and Fascinating Facts about What's All Around Us, by Reader's
Digest. The Reader's Digest Association, Inc.,
1980.

The 2,548 Best Things Anybody Ever Said, by Robert
Byrne. Galahad Books, 1996.

2201 Fascinating Facts, by David Louis. The Ridge
Press, Inc., and Crown Publishers, Inc., 1983.

Uncle John's Bathroom Reader, by the Bathroom Readers' Institute, vols. 1–13. Earthworks Press.

An Underground Education, by Richard Zacks. Anchor
Books, 1997.

Webster's New World Dictionary, Third College Edition. Simon & Schuster, Inc., 1988.

Webster's Unabridged Dictionary, Second Edition.
William Collins & World Publishing Co., Inc.,
1976.

Weird History 101, by John Richard Stephens. Adams
Media Corporation, 1997.

Web Sites

American Bar Association, www.abanet.org

American Medical Association, www.ama-assn.org

Court TV online, www.courttv.com

The Department of Justice's National Criminal Justice
Reference Service,
virlib.ncjrs.org/Statistics.asp

Electric Library, www.elibrary.com

Famous Trials by Doug Linder, www.law.umkc.edu/
faculty/projects/ftrials/ftrials.htm

FindLaw, www.findlaw.com

Lex Antica, members.aol.com/pilgrimjon/
private/LEX/LEX.html

The Paul Revere House, www.paulreverehouse.org

U.S. Department of Labor/Bureau of Labor Statistics,
Occupational Outlook Handbook,
stats.bls.gov/ocohome.htm

U.S. Supreme Court Multimedia Database, The Oyez
Project, Northwestern University,
oyez.nwu.edu

Useless Information,
home.nycap.rr.com/useless/contents.html

Whole Pop Magazine Online, www.wholepop.com

About the Authors

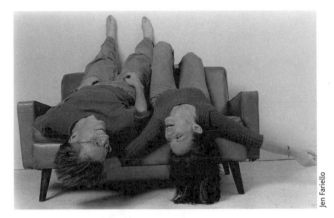

Jen Fariello

Erin Barrett and Jack Mingo have authored twenty books, including *How the Cadillac Got Its Fins, The Couch Potato Guide to Life*, and the bestselling *Just Curious Jeeves.* They have written articles for many major periodicals, including *Salon, The New York Times, The Washington Post,* and *Reader's Digest* and generated more than 30,000 questions for trivia games, and—from their new home in Charlottesville, Virginia—are worried about finding the perfect HMO.

You can contact Erin and Jack at:
ErinBarrett@earthlink.net
JackMingo@earthlink.net